THE GOLDEN FOUNTAIN

The Complete Guide to Urine Therapy

Coen van der Kroon

Translated by
Merilee Dranow

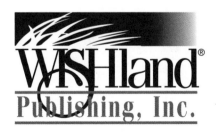

Dutch edition first published in 1993,
copyright © 1993 Coen van der Kroon

English translation by Merilee Dranow, 1996
© Amethyst Books 1996

Reprinted March 1998, March 1999, February 2000

Copyright © Rajesh Bedi, page 34
Photographs in Chapter 4 by Volker Moritz

Designed and typeset by Paperweight

ISBN 0-9632091-5-9

Wishland Publishing, Inc.
Post Office Box 41504
Mesa, Arizona 85274
480-922-8511
Fax 480-443-3386

and in the rest of the world by Gateway Books, The
Hollies, Wellow, Bath BA2 8QJ (tel. 01225835127)

"The human body is the best portrayal of the universe in miniature. Whatever does not exist in the human body cannot be found in the universe, and whatever exists in the universe can be found in the human body."

Mahatma Gandhi

Important Opening Remarks

This book and the therapy it describes are not intended to be a replacement for any other medical treatment which you are receiving or possibly will receive.

The information in this book is based on the author's experiences and on facts as reported in various publications.

Begin treatment of a specific illness only if you consider yourself to be sufficiently informed and, if necessary, professionally supervised.

If you plan to practice urine therapy, proceed with caution. It is of the utmost importance that you are aware of how all natural cures work.

Natural cures work 'from the inside out'. Symptoms which have been suppressed, such as through the use of allopathic medication, can temporarily recur. Healing from the inside out causes the body to detoxify, and can cause severe and sometimes unpleasant reactions.

It is not recommended to practice urine therapy in combination with the use of allopathic medicines or recreational drugs.

The therapy described in this book is meant for those who are willing to take full responsibility for their own health and healing process, and in doing so dare to trust the power of their own body and being.

TABLE OF CONTENTS

FOREWORD
by Swami Pragyamurti Saraswati

When I was first asked to write a foreword to this book, I was delighted – delighted just to be asked and delighted to be able to contribute something to a subject which has been very dear to my heart and an important part of my life for some years. And then I sat down and read the manuscript of this book, and I realized that this is probably the most complete book on Urine Therapy to be published and therefore there was virtually nothing for me to add! Furthermore, it is being published in Britain and will be readily available here. Those of you already interested in the subject will doubtless be familiar with rummaging through dusty piles of books from India or trying to order something a little more up-to-date from the USA!

The history of Amaroli – the lovely Indian name for Urine Therapy – in itself makes for fascinating reading and will surely encourage those who may feel that they are about to embark on something little known and distinctly odd. It belongs to all of us and is as old as time. And you can be completely reassured by the detailed medical and scientific information given in these pages, and the clear instructions for the various practices of Amaroli. I would like to thank Coen van der Kroon for his extensive and painstaking research, which makes the book so valuable.

As a student and teacher of Yoga, I first came across Amaroli in some of the ancient yogic texts, where it is advised as a *sadhana* or spiritual practice, rather than a therapy or cure for various ailments. But I must confess that my first flirtation with it was short and not very sweet! However, about eight years ago the subject reappeared and I started again, this time without any doubts or hesitation.

And yes, it works! I apply fresh urine daily all over my skin and I also drink it two or three times a day. I have also experimented with only taking it once a day and with drinking the entire day's supply, according to my instinctive feelings about my needs. The first benefits I noticed concerned my skin and my greatly increased energy. And that first winter I didn't get a single cold, whereas in the past I had spent months coughing and sniffing. This lead me to think that the urine must be having a positive effect on my immune system, and I continued to experiment with my consumption of the Golden Nectar.

Eventually I introduced Amaroli to some of the students in the Yoga classes I teach for people living with HIV and AIDS, and was amazed at the open-mindedness and enthusiasm with which they greeted it. Since then, many people are now using their urine to great effect, from clearing up skin infections to increasing their T-cells.

Students tell me that for the first time they feel that they themselves are holding the answers to their health and happiness, instead of sitting around waiting for the miracle drug to be invented.

It is this spiritual dimension to Amaroli that I believe to be the most important. By drinking your own urine – thought by many to be disgusting, and if you are HIV+, then lethal as well – a miraculous transformation takes place. Your attitude to yourself changes; you start to really care for yourself, to love yourself. And this is the first vital step towards self-healing, in the fullest sense of the term.

The practice of Amaroli will continue to spread through word of mouth and with the help of excellent books such as this, so I wish you a lot of pleasure and inspiration in reading this book. After all, there is no money to be made from people who manufacture their own medication, particular to the needs of their body and spirit.

HARI OM TAT SAT.

Swami Pragyamurti Saraswati,
London, 26th November 1994.

INTRODUCTION

We all know that drinking urine is healthy and strengthening, yet most of us have forgotten this. After all, we have all done it for nine months. Before it is born, every child floats in amniotic fluid, which consists primarily of urine from the foetus and stimulates our growth. We drink this fluid and then we urinate. We breathe it in and, in doing so, our lungs grow and develop. We are born, and suddenly we consider it to be dirty. And so we stop…?

Nevertheless, I and many others have begun again. I start every day by drinking a glass of morning urine. "Because it is healthy," is my answer to the regularly asked question, "Why?". At first, most people think I am joking. We have all been taught that urine is dirty. How could urine be healthy, let alone help cure illnesses? Well, not everything we have learned is based on the truth.

Urine is not dirty. In fact, we can safely drink it and rub it into our skin. This assertion raises many questions, and rightly so.

Why is urine healthy, and why does it have such a healing effect on every possible illness? In order to answer these questions, we must first consider the concepts of health and healing.

Many people think that the word 'healing' indicates how we can get rid of a physical ailment or illness as quickly as possible. We are cured if a drink gets rid of the common cold, a pill makes the headache disappear or an aspirin suppresses the flu.

However, healing, like life in general, is not so simple. Our body is not the only significant factor – emotions, thoughts and spirituality also influence our health. True health is created when a person is in physical, emotional, mental and spiritual harmony. Only then does our life force flow through us, and we can proceed vigorously through life. This basic truth is usually ignored in our scientifically-oriented society.

In the book *Urine Therapy: It May Save Your Life!*, Dr. Beatrice Bartnett clarifies this principle by comparing it to a rose: We can observe the magnificent form, see the radiant colors and even smell the fresh and delicate scent. This rose is beautiful because it is alive. Without its life force, the rose would be a mere compilation of molecules, nothing more than leaves and petals. We would not see any radiant colors or smell any delicate scents. The difference illustrated here is known as 'life'. Everything around us is full of life: people, animals, plants and even minerals.

Urine also contains life. It is a liquid full of energy, full of life, a fluid that supports and strengthens the life force already present, and regenerates lost life force.

However, urine is not a miracle drug. As mentioned above, health is also dependent upon other factors: nourishment, surroundings, and emotional and mental 'hygiene'. Urine therapy has proved to be a fantastic and versatile aid in the process of healing and becoming whole. It purifies and restores the body and has a revitalizing effect on the spirit and state of mind. It also stimulates independence and freedom: if it works for you, you always have your own doctor and medicine at your side, free of charge. It is no wonder that many people who use urine therapy consider it to be a gift from the gods.

However much urine therapy may seem to be unorthodox and perhaps revolutionary, it does not introduce anything new or original. Urine therapy has been practiced for thousands of years and has merely fallen a bit into obscurity. But all that is changing.

Some time ago, my attention was drawn to two articles in two Dutch national newspapers dealing with research on yogis (holy men) in India who drink their own urine. (This is, incidentally, a good example of a tradition in which urine therapy has been practiced for thousands of years.) The newspaper reports dealt with research into the effects of a stress-reducing hormone, melatonin, found in urine. Both articles were based on the reputable English weekly journal *The New Scientist*. A quote from one of these articles:

"Tense? A glass of morning urine apparently does wonders. But it must be drunk every day. That advice is not from some urine-reader, it is from M. Mills and T. Faunce of the University of Newcastle in Australia."

After reading this article, I contacted the editorial staff of the newspaper and they were interested in an interview. Of course anybody who drinks his own urine is (still) a sensation in a 'civilized' country like the Netherlands where we are supposed to be beyond medieval beliefs and charlatanism. The interviewer was somewhat surprised when I displayed a series of facts and literature demonstrating that drinking urine is neither a medieval practice nor charlatanism – and that the effects go much further than the mere reduction of stress. Urine therapy has been practiced for millennia, and is still being practiced, not only in 'exotic' countries like India but in the United States and Europe as well, and has proved to achieve positive results with all sorts of ailments, from warts and eczema to cancer and AIDS.

The newspaper interview resulted in numerous reactions from the media; since then I have appeared a number of times on Dutch television and radio. Since these various programs have been aired, I have received many reactions. Many people wanted to know specifically how urine therapy could be applied; some had immediately begun and already reported positive results. Others had questions about how they could get over the psychological barrier in order to be able to drink urine, and whether it was not terribly disgusting. And again others were curious as to why I started urine therapy and from where it originates.

I shall begin by telling my personal story about urine therapy – how I came in contact with it and what has followed since then. Like most people who work with urine therapy, I consider my own experiences with and introduction to it to be very important. Thereafter, I began my 'research phase' in which other people's stories (written and verbal testimony) convinced me even more of the miraculous effects of urine therapy.

I hope to answer many questions in this book. Some of the information reported in this book is based on my own experiences with urine therapy, and some is derived from interviews and literature. Therefore, a large part is a collection and compilation of data as reported elsewhere. I have not changed much in texts where I found that the information was clearly represented in the original version, but have more or less reproduced what was already written. The books *Urine Therapy: It May Save Your Life* by Dr. Beatrice Bartnett and *Amaroli* by Dr. Shankardevan Saraswati provided me with a lot of clear, practical suggestions concerning the application of urine therapy.

The information given deals with the various applications of urine, the history of these applications together with instructions, guidelines and advice, the scientific background, and answers to frequently asked questions.

It is up to you to let your own experience convince you. To those who already drink or otherwise use their life water, and to those who decide to do so after reading this book: Cheers, and to your health!

Coen van der Kroon   Amsterdam 1994

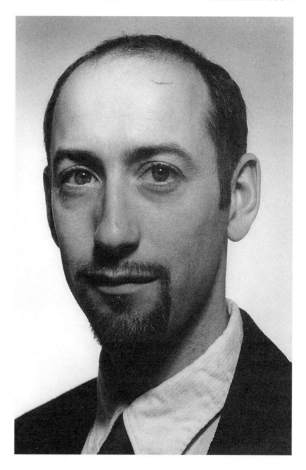

1. GETTING THE TASTE:
An Introduction to Urine Therapy

1.1 My Introduction to Urine Therapy

Many years ago I read an article in the American weekly *Time* in which it was reported that an Indian politician drank a glass of his own urine every day. I found this hard to believe – the thought filled me with disgust. I never would have guessed that some years later I myself would become so deeply involved in the practice of drinking urine. During my quest for information on the background and application of urine therapy, this man's image changed for me from a bizarre man in a magazine to a man whom I visited during my last trip to India.

The man I am referring to is Morarji Desai, former prime minister of India. For years he spoke, in his position as prime minister, about the miraculous therapy which kept him fit and healthy in spite of his advanced age (then almost ninety years old). When I visited him in the spring of 1994, Morarji Desai was ninety-nine years old and still in good health. He drank a glass of urine every day, and massaged and washed himself with it. His skin still looked remarkably radiant and soft. This is how the story in the magazine many years ago literally and figuratively came to life for me.

It was also in India where I was first introduced to urine therapy, although the first book I read there on this subject was written by an Englishman. I found this book in the library of a monastery in the Himalayas. It is called *The Water of Life* and was written in the 1940's by J.W. Armstrong. The book revealed an intriguing fact: by drinking your own urine and massaging yourself with it, you can remain or become perfectly healthy and can recover from the simplest of ailments to the most serious of illnesses. This certainly raised my eyebrows. For years I had been interested in alternative

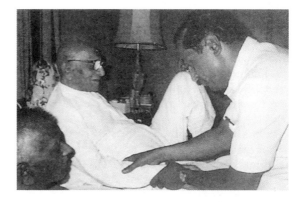

The former Prime Minister of India, Morarji Desai, was a strong propagator of urine therapy. Here, his pulse is being checked by a friend of his, a urine therapist. Morarji Desai died in March 1995, at the age of 100. When I visited him one year before he was still in good health.

medicine, but this miraculous story opened new doors for me. Double doors, that is: besides an enthusiastic interest, I also had a considerable dose of skepticism.

How did this book find its way into my hands? I often ask myself this question. An initially unpleasant experience caused me to get acquainted with urine therapy. The story goes as follows.

Five years ago, I decided to go to India for a few months. I was finished with my studies, and the adventure beckoned. I went to a small monastery ('ashram') in the Himalayas founded by an Indian saint by the name of Babaji of Haidakhan. It was a remote monastery, and one has to walk the last fifteen kilometres through a riverbed to reach it. At first it felt like I had travelled to the end of the world, even though the monastery was named 'the Centre of the World'.

Daily life at the ashram consisted for the most part of hard labor: working in the fields, building, lifting and carrying heavy stones from the riverbed, and all of this at temperatures between 30° and 40° Celsius.

On the second day of my stay there, I had a painful accident which would ultimately lead me to urine therapy. While we were pulling a cart up the side of a mountain, a large stone was knocked loose from a wall and fell one metre onto my left foot. Because I was wearing leather sandals, luckily only my middle toe was seriously injured. I later discovered that it had been broken. At that moment I could see that the flesh, including my toenail, had been ripped off from the upperside of my toe to the bone. An Indian man helped me, and without a moment's hesitation tore off a piece of his shirt and bandaged my toe in order to stop the heavy bleeding.

Back in the monastery, a nurse treated the wound with antiseptic cream and re-bandaged my toe. Although the wound was treated and re-bandaged daily, the pain increased and the toe appeared to get worse and worse. With a serious wound in the tropics,

it is definitely a good idea to seek proper care. An infection can have unpleasant consequences, and wounds heal quite slowly. After a week, I started to worry because my condition worsened, and people started warning me about possible complications, such as gangrene.

At that time I happened to be talking with a woman, also Dutch, who advised me to wind a cloth soaked in my own urine around my toe. My initial reaction was disgust – urine is dirty, so how could it help heal a wound? Even so, I later felt that I should at least try it – the situation could not get any worse. In addition, this woman had in the meantime told me more about urine therapy, and she had also given me the book *The Water of Life* from the library at the monastery. I finally plucked up the courage to try it.

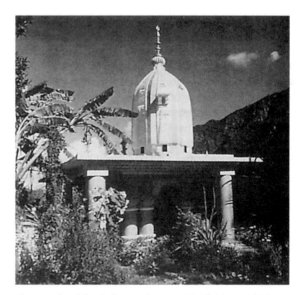

The temple of the Babaji-Ashram in Haidakhan, a little village in the foothills of the Himalayas.

The following day while I was reading this book (with a cloth soaked in my own urine wrapped around my toe), I oscillated between my aversion to urine and the persuasive contents of the book I was reading.

It was stated in the book that, by drinking your own urine and massaging yourself with it, you could cure various wounds, ailments and illnesses. In the first half of this century, Armstrong, the author of the book, promoted the use of urine therapy. Although his doctors had offered him little hope of recovering, Armstrong cured himself of tuberculosis with the help of urine therapy. Thereafter he began helping and advising others. He successfully treated hundreds of patients, many of whom were suffering from life-threatening illnesses such as tuberculosis and cancer. Armstrong recorded the results of these treatments. *The Water of Life* has since become a standard work in the application of urine therapy, both here in the West as well as in India.

At that time however I still could not imagine that I could drink my own urine without a strong aversion, and yet I had a feeling that what was written in that book was true. Quite apart from my intuition, I also have a fairly academically inclined mind, and the combination of the two stimulated me at least to research and test this whole business thoroughly!

The experience with my toe was what really persuaded me to do this. After three days the wound was completely clean, the swelling was gone and the pain considerably reduced. On the fourth day, radiant, new, pink skin appeared under the wound tissue. A few days thereafter, the wound was almost completely healed and a new nail had even started to grow. It was obvious that something quite unusual had happened here: in a tropical climate, it normally takes at least three weeks under the most favorable conditions for such a deep wound to close up and heal. Within a week, the combination of my own experience and reading that book had won me over. I

was keen to know more!

But where could I learn more? Who knew about this therapy in our Western culture? Research and university libraries did not yield any information. The year following my return from India, I drank my urine in the morning from time to time, but there were also times when I thought, "What am I doing this for? Could I be going too far in my belief and trust in something so bizarre?" Whenever I caught a cold or the flu, I fasted for a day or two on urine and water, and quickly felt better, but, even then, I would question whether this also would have happened without drinking my urine.

A year later I was travelling in the United States. While shopping at a bookstore specializing in spiritual awareness and alternative medicine, I suddenly came across a small, blue book entitled *The Miracles of Urine Therapy*. I was pleasantly surprised! I had been looking for this book without even knowing it existed. It was a recently published work by a Swiss-American natural doctor who had even established a Water of Life Institute in America. The book contained practical information about urine therapy, as well as texts from various cultures and religions which show that the origin of this therapy is centuries old, both in the Far East and here in the West. My trip to the United States had been worthwhile, if only for this discovery.

Back in the Netherlands, I plunged into my research on urine therapy with renewed enthusiasm. I contacted the Water of Life Institute in the United States and received more information from them, specifically on the scientific background of urine therapy. From this information I learned, for instance, that many separate components of urine are used in cosmetic products, without our being aware of it.

Soon after this, I came across a cosmetic product in which urea was processed. Apart from water, urea is the main component of urine, so you can imagine that this provided a wonderful topic for conversation: you often 'use' urine without even being aware of it.

As a result of the increasing number of questions I received each time I told my story, I decided to start giving lectures. Several people in the audience related their own experiences with urine therapy, once again a sign that it was not as obscure as I had initially assumed. Many people knew it was once used for chillblains and for disinfecting wounds.

For most of the audience, though, all this was completely new. For them, the first question was always: "If urine is a waste product, isn't it un-healthy to drink it?" Since then I have found that my most important task has been to break down this psychological barrier. Urine is not dirty. Urine is, in fact, a clean substance: it is sterile, consists for the most part of water and for the remaining part of harmless and often even beneficial substances.

I began to enjoy telling people about this 'shocking' therapy and seeing the various reactions, which ranged from total disgust to instant enthusiasm. Several times, people were so keen on the idea that they immediately began the next morning. Others believe in it, but cannot bring themselves to take even a sip of it. Whatever the reaction, though, the topic of conversation often leads to a good laugh, in itself very healthy.

I decided to return to India in order to look for people who worked with urine therapy. After staying for a few weeks in the same monastery I had visited earlier, I went to New Delhi in the hope of finding more literature on this subject in a small bookstore I knew of there. After digging around in enormous, chaotic piles of books, I was delighted to see the owner appear with two books on urine therapy, one of which had recently been published by someone in Bombay. Considering that I already had an address there, it seemed clear that this was to be my next port of call.

I also had an address in Baroda, and so I made a stopover there on my way to Bombay. Indian cities are large, chaotic and swarming with people. The inhabitants often do not know the names of the streets and the thousands of alleys in the city – and this also goes for the rikshaw- and taxi-drivers. It took me two full days of rambling around in this city devoid of tourists in order to find the address I was seeking. On top of that, when I finally got there, the door of the house was locked. A crowd quickly gathered around to find out what I, a Western foreigner, was doing there. In the broken English conversation that followed with the 'street-elders', I finally had to acknowledge that my efforts had been in vain: the man I sought, who offered advice on urine therapy, was travelling at that time and I could not find out when he would be back.

I therefore decided to move on to Bombay, a day's travelling by train, where I had much more success. I met with three enthusiastic urine therapists, including the founder and chairman of the Water of Life Foundation India, Dr. G.K. Thakkar. Dr. Thakkar was also a lawyer and tax consultant. These were his original two professions, but, throughout the years, the number of people that came to him for advice on the subject of urine therapy had steadily grown. Three professions are stated on his business card: lawyer, tax consultant and urine therapist, a combination which would certainly perplex people in the West!

Dr. Thakkar sees his 'patients' at his office in one of the busy, overcrowded streets of Bombay. At the end of the day he receives patients with all sorts of complaints, from the common cold to cancer. They get free advice and consultations from him while he works on complicated tax papers. Dr. Thakkar himself suffered from amoebic dysentery and eczema for twenty years before he was introduced to urine therapy five years ago. Like most other Indian urine therapists with whom I have spoken or corresponded, Dr. Thakkar talks about urine therapy as if it were a gift from God. He has since given lectures at various international conferences on natural medicine. When I visited him, he invited me to attend his consultations for a few days, which I of course did with much interest and pleasure.

I also found some more books on urine therapy in a bookstore in Bombay. The amount of information and literature I collected had thus grown considerably after my visit to this bookstore. Together with the copies of newspaper clippings and a list of all the urine therapists in India which I had collected, I now had access to the most important written information available on this subject. It was a successful expedition – not only from a research point of view, but also because my regular use of urine therapy helped me to remain healthy for the whole trip in India without the usual pills and injections Westerners are normally advised to take.

Satisfied with my research, I concluded my second adventure in India, and in the spring of 1992 I returned to the Netherlands.

A few weeks after my return, I 'achieved' a new success. People around me told me that my hair had become fuller and that the bald patch at the back of my head had practically disappeared. I had not noticed it yet, but I then realized that my experiment had yielded good results: The fact is, at the beginning of my trip to India, I had begun massaging four-day old urine into my scalp and had maintained this fairly consistently during my six-week tour. I was curious to see if this would have any effect, but to be honest, I did not believe too much in this treatment. This experience, however, added to my faith in the regenerative powers of urine.

A little later, in the summer of 1992, I was approached a number of times by the media, which resulted in a few interviews on television, radio and in the newspapers. More and more people asked me for advice; others telephoned me to relate their own experiences. I got in touch with Carmen Thomas, a woman who worked on German radio (WDR); she had done a program four years earlier about urine therapy. Since then, she had been receiving dozens of letters every week with experiences, stories and positive reactions. She also recently published a book in Germany about the many

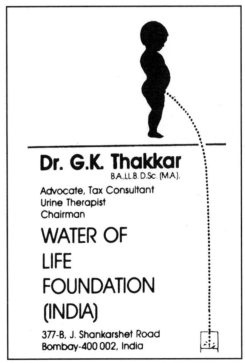

Business card of Dr. Thakkar.

applications of urine, *Ein ganz besonderer Saft – Urin* ('A Very Special Juice – Urine'), which in the meantime has become an absolute bestseller.

In her book, Carmen Thomas discusses the various ways urine was formerly used, specifically in Germany, and is still used today. Just one example is the use of urine as a remedy for illnesses. The book contains dozens of personal stories from people in Germany who have somehow or other either benefited from the use of urine or have been cured of their illness or ailments. But that is not all. The other possible uses of urine are also addressed. For example, urine was often used in the manufacturing and care of textiles and as an aid in the painting of fabrics. Urine was also used as a detergent in ancient Rome, and much later in Germany, urine was collected for the village or city laundries by the so-called 'Seck-Hannes', which literally translated means 'Piss-Hans'. Urine was also used in a variety of other branches: for hardening iron, baking bread, making cheese and treating leather, to mention a few.

At one point I heard that a conference on urine therapy would be held in India: *The First All India Conference on Urine Therapy*. I immediately felt that I simply had to be there. In February 1993, I arrived in India and travelled on to Goa, where the conference would take place. The location turned out to be a beautiful temple complex in the middle of an exotic landscape. Some two hundred people from India were present, including doctors, urine therapists who had been working with urine for more than twenty years, people who were being or had been treated, and those who simply wanted to know more.

At the conference a great deal of attention was given to the experiences people had gained in treating themselves or others. At the same time, however, it seemed there was not enough documented material on all these experiences, and that this would be necessary in the future for more scientific research. A number of people questioned the reliability of the literature on urine therapy. After all, the literature is full of 'miraculous recoveries', but cases in which urine therapy does not work seem to be omitted.

It is important to develop a more scientifically grounded approach. Even though I am personally convinced

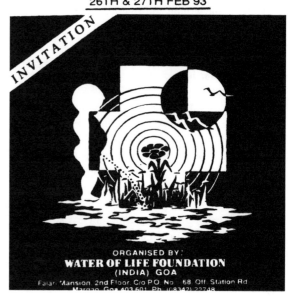

The invitation for the Shivambu Kalpa (Urine Therapy) conference in Goa, India, in 1993.

of the positive effects of urine therapy and have seen very impressive results, I consider it important to present an honest and complete summary of what is presently known to those who have not yet experienced it – certainly those in our modern, scientific society who first need 'hard evidence' before they are willing to risk trying something new.

At any rate, the conference in Goa set things in motion, and plans were made to organize an international event. And it really seems that all around the world interest in this simple and effective therapy is rapidly growing.

In the meantime, I will continue working enthusiastically to promote and make this exceptional therapy known. To be honest, I also see it as a gift from God (or whatever you choose to call it) that I am able to work with urine therapy.

1.2 A Brief Introduction to the Principles of Urine Therapy

Before going on to the chapters which discuss the history and application of urine therapy, I shall briefly discuss the composition of urine, what urine therapy is and how it works.

So, what does urine consist of? 95% of urine is water, 2°% consists of urea and the remaining 2°% is a mixture of minerals, salt, hormones and enzymes. Only urea, the substance after which urine is named, can be poisonous when present in very large amounts in the blood. However, this is irrelevant in the practice of drinking urine, as urine is not immediately put back in the bloodstream. In the small amounts urea gets back into the body, it is purifying, clears up excess mucus and has a number of specific, very useful effects which will be discussed later in this book. Furthermore, urine is entirely sterile after secretion and has an antiseptic effect.

We are talking here about urine from the point of view of somebody who follows a reasonably healthy diet, and who does not use drugs or allopathic medicines. Urine therapy is a method based upon the principle of 'natural cycles'. As long as we do not interfere chemically with the body's natural cycle, the body produces urine which is perfectly suitable for recycling. If you ingest a great deal of chemical substances – and these days all kinds of processed food contain chemicals – part of this will end up in the urine, in which case the composition of the urine changes. Normally, however, urine is a healthy substance which contains healthy, harmless components.

Urine therapy is a natural medicine. Natural medicines work with natural and harmless therapies, and focus on the whole person. Natural medicines also focus on stimulating the self-regulating power of the body and encouraging personal responsibility for health and well-being. The ancient Greek doctor Hippocrates (circa 500 B.C.), one of the founders of Western medicine, often referred to this self-regulating power of the human organism. In the medical world, this power was later referred to as *vix medicatrix naturae* ('the healing power of nature').

In the past few decades, the medical world has regularly been confronted with illnesses and symptoms which are related to a failing defense or immune system. The self-healing power and the immune system are related. Nowadays many doctors acknowledge the importance of research on the immune system and the mechanisms of self-healing. This has led to new approaches within medical science and urine therapy could provide very interesting areas of research as far as this field is concerned.

Urine therapy is indeed natural and harmless and can thus be regarded as belonging to the realms of natural medicine. Those who practice this therapy believe that it has an intensely positive effect on the self-healing power of the human body.

As said before, urine therapy is based upon the existence of a natural cycle. Some cycles take place more quickly than others, but the cycle in general is the foundation of all life. If we let nature run her course, there will be no waste, and a disturbed equilibrium will always come back into balance. Just as we are capable of disturbing a natural equilibrium, we can also do our part in helping nature recover her balance. In order to support such a recovering of balance, we are equipped with a wonderful, natural 'house pharmacy': our own urine provides us with a swift and safe method for using the powers of the natural cycle.

What exactly are the effects of urine therapy? We come back to and comprehensively deal with this question in Chapter 5, including the most recent scientific information on urine therapy. Briefly, if urine is ingested and rubbed into the skin, it purifies blood and tissues, provides useful nutrients and sends the body a signal about what is in or out of balance. The effects of intensive application of urine therapy in which a person fasts exclusively on urine and water are described by Armstrong in his book *The Water of Life* as follows:

"Urine, on being taken into the body, is filtered; it becomes purer and purer even in the course of one day's living upon it, plus tap-water, if required. First, it cleanses, then frees from obstruction and finally rebuilds the vital organs and passages after they have been wasted by the ravages of disease. In fact it rebuilds not only the lungs, pancreas, liver, brain, heart, etc., but also repairs the linings of brain and bowel and other linings, as has been demonstrated in the case of many 'killing' diseases, such as consumption of the intestines and the worst form of colitis. In fine, it accomplishes what fasting merely on water or fruit juices (as some naturopaths advocate) can never achieve."

(From: *The Water of Life*, J.W. Armstrong, Health Science Press, London 1971, p. 26)

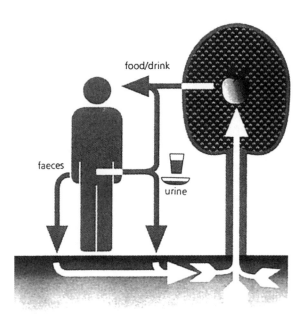

food/drink

faeces

urine

Everything consists of natural cycles. Whatever leaves our bodies, is taken in again in one way or the other. Urine therapy is nothing but a health-promoting variety of this system of natural cycles.

Armstrong uses natural metaphors in order to illustrate the effects of urine therapy. Nature knows how to take care of herself; there is much to learn from her. In order to remain in balance, she makes use of an economically and ecologically perfect system called recycling, in which nothing is wasted. For example, leaves fall from the trees in autumn. The leaves decay, and the remains slowly sink into the earth. The tree feeds on these same substances the next season. If we let the fallen leaves remain on the ground instead of raking them away, the trees yield a larger and better crop the next season.

The cycle of water is another example. The sun evaporates water, and this consequently forms clouds. Some time later the clouds release water, usually in the form of rain or snow. Back on the ground, water cleanses the earth and serves as a nutrient, until it returns to a reservoir and is evaporated again.

Similar cycles also exist within ourselves. Our blood has its own cycle; the heart pumps it through the body. The most important function of blood is to transport oxygen and nutrients to every cell in the body, and it passes through the liver and kidneys on its way.

One of the liver's most important functions is detoxification of the blood. The liver removes poisonous substances from the blood and either stores them or secretes them into the gall-bladder. In the latter case, the poisonous substances end up as bile in the intestinal canal. They then leave the body in the form of defecation. After the blood is detoxified by the liver, it flows to the kidneys. This is, of course, a simplified explanation.

The kidneys' most important function consists of balancing out all elements in the blood. They remove all superfluous vital substances from the blood, and filter out a surplus of water. This water and the vital substances consequently form urine. For example, at any given moment, the body can absorb only a certain amount of vitamin C. Any surplus vitamin C in the bloodstream is at that moment unusable and consumes energy; after all, it has to be transported. This is why the body removes the surplus of vitamin C through the kidneys.

A second example: In order to activate an enzyme, a second co-enzyme is necessary. This co-enzyme is usually a mineral or vitamin brought into the body with our food. The co-enzyme activates and transports

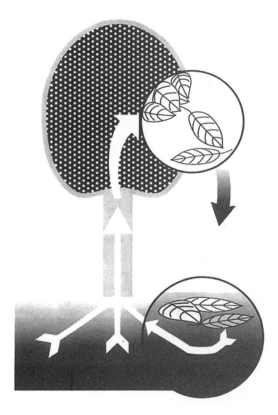

A natural cycle: trees grow best when they feed on their own fallen leaves.

the enzymes to the proper location in the body. Even if our body produces more than enough enzymes, it cannot function optimally if our food does not contain enough nutrients, and thus co-enzymes. In order to save energy and bring the blood into balance, the kidneys remove unused enzymes from the blood. The same goes for hormones, minerals and other substances. It is clear that urine is full of vital elements, which can hardly be called waste products.

The harmful waste products which nonetheless can be found in urine are often the result of unhealthy eating and drinking habits. This includes consuming products which contain chemical additives and radiation, alcohol, nicotine, caffeine or indigestible fats. As previously mentioned, it is therefore advisable to follow a healthy and non-toxic diet while applying urine therapy. If you do so, your urine will also remain healthy and non-toxic. After all, no substance which has not earlier been consumed will appear in the urine. This does not mean that consuming toxic products excludes the use of urine therapy, but it may make it less effective.

If a pathological process is in progress, the body may produce poisonous substances. If these substances, or part of these, end up in the urine, drinking urine can have a homeopathic or isopathic effect. These substances are not foreign to the body, and can fulfill an important role in restoring the natural balance. This usually concerns relatively small amounts, unless the kidneys, bladder or urinary passages are inflamed, in which case some caution is required. In those cases urine therapy can be applied by placing a few drops of urine on or under the tongue or by means of a homeopathic dilution. You can read all about the practical applications of urine therapy – possibilities and limitations – in Chapter 4 of this book.

To repeat, the liver detoxifies the blood and secretes the waste products in the intestinal canal. The kidneys,

as mentioned above, keep the vital substances and the water level in balance.

So urine is actually filtered blood. When fresh, it merely contains substances and elements found in the bloodstream. Substances which at one point were an integral part of your blood, and therefore of yourself, shortly thereafter become your urine. So, actually, you are ingesting nothing more or less than yourself.

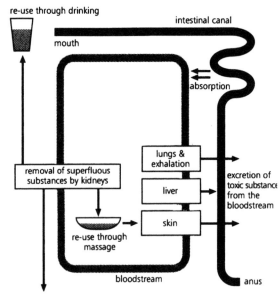

A schematic and simplified representation of the excretion system of the human body: liver, lungs and skin excrete the toxic substances from the body; the kidneys filter superfluous substances from the blood. In this way the kidneys guarantee an optimal equilibrium of the elements the blood is composed of. Taking these substances into the body again, e.g. by drinking urine or massaging it into the skin, creates the possibility to use them once again. In this way we just make use of a natural cycle, offered to us by our own bodies.

2. THE WATER OF LIFE:
The History of Urine Therapy in the West

2.1 The Use of Urine in Ancient Europe

Urine therapy is the most primitive, original and simple form of homeopathy or isopathy. Although this natural healing method is still widely used in India, urine therapy is not only an Eastern tradition. In fact the use of urine as medicine in one form or another can be found in many medical traditions of people or tribes which are still in close contact with nature. I recently heard a story from a native North American who told that he has used urine therapy his whole life in order to purify his body and soul periodically. He had learned this from his parents and grandparents. Gypsies and Eskimos still use urine as medicine. Eskimo women often use urine as shampoo; it gives hair extra body and a beautiful shine.

Also many people in the modern Western world of Europe and America are familiar with the use of urine in treating warts, chillblained hands and feet, and as a disinfectant for minor wounds.

The use of urine is thus also rooted in the European tradition. Doctors in ancient Greece reportedly used urine for healing wounds. In book 28 of his *Naturalis Historia* ('Natural History'), the Roman author C. Plinius Secundus discusses the medicinal use of urine in the treatment of wounds, dog and snake bites, skin diseases, eye infections, burns and scars. Although only a few sources in Western history can be found which discuss the use of urine as medicine, a number of sources describe other possible applications of urine. A number of examples are discussed below.

Urine was used in ancient Rome for washing and dying textiles. Urine was centrally collected by so-called laundries, as it is an excellent detergent and cleanser. Large stone jugs for collecting urine were placed on street corners. Urine was so important during the time of the Roman Empire that, according to the author Suetonius, Emperor Vespasian levied taxes on every drop collected in public toilets and the urine jars. Urine was therefore a commodity, and the emperor Vespasian wanted to get his share of this lucrative business. The 'urine-traders' thought the urine tax was unfair: the work they performed was oppressive because the old urine stank so badly. Vespasian was not interested in their objections. *"Money does not stink"* (*pecunia non olet*) was his answer to their complaints, and is the origin of this well-known expression. Even today in Paris, a public urinal is known as a *Vespasienne*.

It is actually quite logical that urine was used in the laundering industry. Chemical research has demonstrated that when urine (particularly the ammonia found in urine) is mixed with fat, a white soap is spontaneously created. This partly explains why urine is so effective in keeping skin and hair clean and healthy, without the use of soap or shampoo.

Urine has also been used in the textile industry in Northern Europe, particularly as detergent. I have already referred to the collecting of urine by city laundries in German villages and cities. Another interesting example can be found in Tilburg, The Netherlands where a statue by the name of 'The Bottle-Pisser' is displayed. A short history of the name 'The Bottle-Pisser' is given on the back side of a postcard of this statue:

"Tilburg formerly had a farming population, which lived in poverty. In the Middle Ages, the Tilburg farmer started spinning wool from his own sheep and wove it on a homemade loom in his living room. He kept part of the wool for his family and sold the rest. In this way, the wool industry, which made Tilburg great, became a domestic industry. Later, small factories were established where wage laborers worked for a few cents per hour. The material was refined in a particular way, known as splashing and milling. Ammonia, found in urine, was necessary in order to mill and paint the wool. And so the laborers were paid to bring their own urine to work. Some laborers received a payment of up to thirty to forty guilders annually for their urine. It is said that Monday's urine was not acceptable, due to the high percentage of alcohol it contained. And so the Tilburg population was named 'Bottle-Pissers.'"

Yet another use for urine can be found in the Celtic culture of the Druids. The older Druids periodically went into a trance in order to be able to perform their rituals. To do so, they made use of so-called 'magic mushrooms', mushrooms which induced a hallucinatory state. However, these mushrooms also contained poisonous substances which could inhibit the hallucinatory process and cause damage to the liver. They therefore had young men eat the mushrooms first so their livers could filter out the mushrooms' poisonous substances. The hallucinatory substances, in themselves not poisonous, remained in the blood and were urinated out of the body some time later. The older Druids then drank the urine, and in this way safely reached an altered state of consciousness!

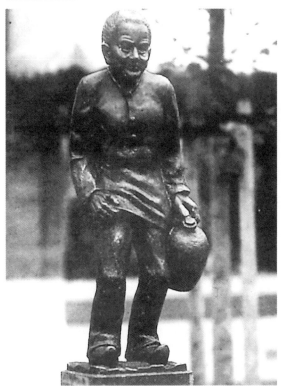

Statue of a so-called 'Bottle-Pisser' from the Dutch city of Tilburg.

This tradition was also known by the Finno-Ugric tribes in Siberia. In the book *Plants of the Gods*, a passage on the hallucinogenic mushroom 'amanita muscaria' (Fly Agaric) includes a reference to drinking urine:

"These Siberian mushroom users had no other intoxicants, until the Russians introduced alcohol. They dried the mushrooms in the sun and ingested them either alone or as an extract in water, reindeer milk, or the juice of several sweet plants. When the mushroom was swallowed as a solid, it was first moistened in the mouth, or a woman rolled it in her mouth into a moistened pellet for the men to swallow. The ceremonial use of the Fly Agaric developed a ritualistic practice of urine-drinking, since these tribesmen learned that the psychoactive principles of the mushroom pass through the body unmetabolized or in the form of still active metabolites – most unusual for hallucinogenic compounds in plants. An early account, referring to the Koryak, reported that "they pour water on some of these mushrooms and boil them. They then drink the liquor, which intoxicates them; the poorer sort, who cannot afford to lay in a store of the mushrooms, post themselves on these occasions round the huts of the rich and watch the opportunity of the guests coming down to make water and then hold a wooden bowl to receive the urine, which they drink off greedily, as having still some virtue of the mushroom in it, and by this way, they also get drunk.""

(From: *Plants of the Gods; Their Sacred Healing and Hallucinogenic Powers*, Evans Schultes, R. & Hofmann, A., Healing Arts Press, Rochester Vermont 1992, p. 83)

George Andrews mentions in his book *Drugs and Magic* (1975) that the reindeer hunters of the Middle Anadyr, Siberia, used Fly Agaric mushrooms and when there was a shortage of the mushrooms they would drink cupfuls of each other's urine without inhibition to prolong the effect.

2.2 Medical Use of Urine in the Last Centuries

Throughout history, urine has played a part in the alchemist tradition. Nowadays urine still plays a role in the preparation and use of medicines produced on an alchemical basis. The well-known Dutch aurologist and alchemist Jelle Veeman has spoken many times about the significance of urine in this context. The following fragment illustrates the use of urine by so-called alchemists:

"Phosphorus was discovered in 1669, by Brandt, a Hamburg chemist who was looking for the philosophers' stone. He believed that the metal could be transmuted into gold by mixing it with the extract of urine. Using this method, he obtained a luminous substance that burned with an intensity such as had never been seen before. For a long time phosphorus was obtained by vigorously heating the residue of evaporating urine in an earth retort the neck of which was submerged in water. Today it is extracted from the bones of animals, which contain phosphoric acid and lime."

(From: *Like Water for Chocolate*, Laura Esquivel, Anchor Books Doubleday, New York 1992)

Since approximately 1700, a number of sources explicitly refer to the healing effect of urine. A dentist in Paris in the eighteenth century praised urine as an extremely valuable mouthwash, and French and German doctors used cow-urine in the eighteenth century to control and cure jaundice, rheumatic disorders, gout, dropsy, sciatica and asthma.

Johann Heinrich Zedler is quoted in the *Grossen Vollständigen Universallexikon* (1747), in which he offers the following tips concerning the use of urine as medicine:

> "Useful substances can be found in human as well as animal urine... Human urine has strengthening and curative characteristics concerning many deficiencies:

> "For example, a mixture of potato- and sulphur-powder, mixed with heated, old urine helps against hair loss. One should rub this mixture into the scalp; this slows down loss of hair (calf's gall can be added if necessary).

> "One can best heal injuries to the eyes with honey dissolved in the lightly boiled urine from a young man. One should wash the eyes as often as possible with this fluid.

> "All kinds of throat inflammation can be helped by gargling with urine to which a bit of saffron has been added.

> "Trembling hands and knees can be helped by washing and rubbing one's own warm urine into the skin directly after one has urinated.

> "In the beginning stages of dropsy, one should drink one's own morning urine on an empty stomach for a prolonged period of time. This also helps against jaundice."

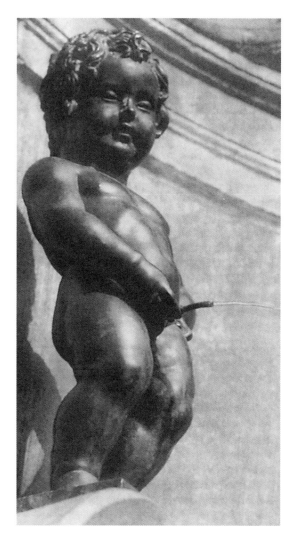

'Manneke Pis', a playful symbol of urine in Europe.

In his book, Armstrong quotes the English book *One Thousand Notable Things*, which was published in England, Scotland and Ireland at the end of the eighteenth century. A number of quotations are given below:

"An universal and excellent remedy for all distempers inward and outward. Drink your own water in the morning nine days together and it cures the scurvy, makes the body lightsome and cheerful.

"It is good against the dropsy and jaundice, drunk as before (stated).

"Wash your ears with it warm and it is good against deafness, noises and most other ailments in the ears.

"Wash your eyes with your own water and it cures sore eyes and clears and strengthens the sight.

"Wash and rub your hands with it and it takes away numbness, chaps and sores and makes the joints limber.

"Wash any green wound with it and it is an extraordinary good thing.

"Wash any part that itches and it takes it (the itch) away.

"Wash the fundament and it is good against piles and other sores."

(From: *The Water of Life*, J.W. Armstrong, Health Science Press, London 1971, p. 13.)

This fragment indicates how versatile the applications of urine were seen to be: from harmless itching to serious conditions, such as gangrene.

Other notable fragments on the application and characteristics of urine can be found in the book *Salmon's English Physician*, published in 1695. A number of quotations from this book quoted in *The Water of Life* follow below:

"Urine is taken from human kind and most four-footed animals; but the former is that which is chiefly used in Physick and Chemistry. It is the serum or watery part of the blood, which being diverted by the emulgent arteries to the veins is there separated, and by the ferment of the parts, converted into urine... Man's or woman's urine is hot, dry, dissolving, cleansing, discussing, resists putrefaction; used inwardly against obstructions of the liver, spleen, gall, as also against the Dropsie, Jaundice, Stoppage of the terms in women, the Plague and all manner of malign fevers.

"Outwardly (applied) it cleanses the skin and softens it by washing it therewith, especially being warm, or new made. Cleanses, heals and dries up wounds, though made with poisoned weapons. Cures dandruff, scurf, and bathed upon the pulses, cools the heat of fevers. Is excellent against trembling, numbness and the palsy, and bathed upon the region of the spleen, urine eases the pains thereof.

"The virtues of the volatile salts of urine. It powerfully absorbs acids and destroys the very root of most diseases in human bodies. It opens all obstructions of... Veins, Mysentery and Womb, purifies the whole mass of Blood and Humors cures... Caclexia... Rheumatism and Hypochondriac diseases, and is given with admirable success in Epilepsies, Vertigoes, Apoplexies, Convulsions, Lythargies, Migraine, palsies, Lameness, Numbness, loss of the use of

limbs, atrophies, vapors, fits of the mother, and most cold and moist diseases of the head, brain, nerves, joints and womb. (Leucorrhoea should be added to this list.)

"It opens obstructions of the veins and urinary passages, dissolves tartarous coagulations in those parts, breaks and expels stone and gravel.

"It is a specific remedy against Dysuria, Ischuria and all obstructions of Urine whatsoever."

(From: *The Water of Life*, J.W. Armstrong, Health Science Press, London 1971, p. 13-15.)

This fragment also indicates how versatile the author found the application of urine to be: many different illnesses and ailments are mentioned. Besides, he explains that urine is simply a component of the blood and that it is purifying and prevents decay and putrefaction.

2.3   20th Century Developments of Urine Therapy

Armstrong also quotes an article from a contemporary scholar, Professor Jean Rostand, which discusses the biological importance of hormones and the fact that these can be found in large quantities in human urine. A passage from this article reads as follows:

"A recent discovery regarding the activity of hormones has completely revolutionized their study – viz., that certain of them filter through the kidney to pass out in the urine. Multiple hypophysical hormones, the hormones of the adrenal and hormones of the sexual glands, have been found in normal urine... The discovery of hormone-urinology has had far-reaching consequences. Urine provides a practically unlimited quantity of basic matter... From the therapeutic point of view it is possible to envisage the use of these human hormones as apparently capable of exercising great power over the human organism..."

(From: *The Water of Life*, J.W. Armstrong, Health Science Press, London 1971, p. 15.)

It is obvious that this man was far ahead of his time: scientists have only recently started research on the hormonal effects of urine. Later in this book, I shall discuss this aspect of urine therapy in more detail.

Dr. T. Wilson Deachman, another scholar from the beginning of this century, recognized the enormous value of urine and the intelligence of the body as a self-healing organism. Apparently other doctors did not listen to him. This is what he wrote about urine:

"As the urine content varies according to the pathological state of the patient, its use is indicated in all forms of disease except those caused by traumatism (broken limbs) or those that are of a mechanical nature. It saves the physician from the mistake that is made in selecting the indicated remedy from three thousand drugs or more... What cannot be cured by the forces of the body cannot be cured by the forces outside the body."

(From: *The Water of Life*, J.W. Armstrong, Health Science Press, London 1971, p. 156)

Armstrong quotes another fragment, a report from *Doctors, Disease and Health* by Cyril Scott about a certain Mr. Baxter, who was Armstrong's patient for a short period of time:

"Mr. Baxter, who lived to a ripe old age, declaring that he had cured himself of a cancerous growth by applying his own urine in the form of compresses, and by drinking his own urine neat. He further declared that he had cured himself of other complaints by these simple means. Mr. Baxter contended that urine is the finest antiseptic that exists, and, having made this discovery, he formed the daily habit of drinking three tumblers full as a prophylactic against disease. He maintained that if autogenous urine is taken in this way, the more innocuous it becomes. He applied it to his eyes as a strengthening lotion, and used it, after shaving, for his complexion. He also advocated its external use for wounds, swellings, boils, etc."

(From: *The Water of Life*, J.W. Armstrong, Health Science Press, London 1971, p. 17.)

Although Armstrong must have been quite pleased with this handful of quotations from scholars, he realized that the powerful medical world entertained other ideas. Even so, he was exceptionally persistent in his conviction and enthusiasm concerning urine therapy, probably because through urine therapy, he cured himself of tuberculosis which had been declared 'incurable'.

Armstrong began urine therapy after a long and agonizing journey in which doctor after doctor proved unable to cure him of his symptoms. On the contrary, his condition only worsened. He decided to try urine therapy for two reasons. First of all, a quotation from the Bible stimulated his curiosity: *"Drink water from your own cistern, flowing water from your own well."* (*The Book of Proverbs* 5:15) Secondly, he had childhood memories of his mother smearing urine on his face which was swollen from a bee sting, and of his grandfather treating animals with urine.

Armstrong is unclear as to whether this quotation from the Bible should be interpreted as he has, but he does claim it to be the source of inspiration for his beginning a forty-five day fast based exclusively on urine and water. He combined this fast with massaging urine into his skin, based upon what he found in another passage in the Bible, the *Gospel of Matthew* 6:17-18: *"But when you fast, anoint your head and wash your face,..."* He found that fasting was much easier and more pleasant if he also massaged himself with (old) urine.

After his own successful experience, Armstrong treated hundreds of people with urine therapy. Only after a number of years, and at the explicit request of those he had treated, did he write a book about his own experiences and knowledge. This is the previously mentioned and praised book *The Water of Life*. This book was and continues to be a great source of inspiration for everyone who works with urine therapy, both in the West and in the East.

As mentioned above, Armstrong realized all too well that his message was not in keeping with the prevailing scientific dogma. Unfortunately, his worthwhile results did not stimulate other doctors in England to delve into this subject.

Nonetheless, in other countries several attempts have been made by doctors to bring urine treatments to a scientific level. They worked with urine injections which were first performed with the invention of the hypodermic needle and syringe. This method was applied in Europe as well as in the United States, which is apparent from *The Physiological Memoirs of Surgeon-General Hammond, U.S. Army* (1863) in which reference is made to this method. These days few doctors give urine injections; only Heilpraktiker (natural doctors) in Germany use this method regularly. They specifically consider urine injections to be a worthwhile method of treating illnesses related to allergies. This application of urine therapy was recently highlighted on a German commercial television broadcasting station in which several people with allergies were shown injecting themselves with urine.

The medical interest in urine and its components increased around the beginning of this century, particularly in Germany. Experiments were conducted on injecting urine, and the results were positive.

The German physician Dr. Herz was an enthusiastic proponent of this method and, in 1930, he wrote a book reporting his experiences (*Die Eigenharnbehandlung*, 'Auto-Urine Treatment'). Although scientists and clinics were initially interested in his work, his research came to a halt, since the German government at the time tightened the veins on scientific research. Even so, a number of doctors kept practicing this therapy.

In the 1940's, doctors in Germany gave urine-enemas to children exposed to measles or smallpox. Those treated with urine-enemas came down with a milder form of these illnesses. The German physician Dr. Martin Krebs wrote *Der menschliche Harn als Heilmittel* ('Human Urine as Medicine'), a book about the application and results of urine therapy with children. Martin Krebs was a fervent follower of Dr. Herz.

In 1965, Dr. Edam from Germany recommended urine therapy as the most effective treatment for morning sickness during pregnancy, and advised the larger university hospitals to try this method instead of the frequent use of medication. He maintained that no side effects had been diagnosed, and he hoped more doctors would take an interest in this therapy.

Scientists also began to research the effectiveness of the separate components of urine. Hundreds of research reports have been published on the component urea, apart from water the main component of urine. In Chapter 5, the importance of urea, a simple breakdown-product of proteins, regarding the effects of urine therapy is discussed in more detail.

Research has been conducted into the possible medicinal effects of urine's individual components, such as the hormone specimens obtained from pregnant women's urine. Under the motto 'mothers for mothers', urine is collected from pregnant women and processed into a hormone product for those women who have difficulty getting pregnant. Another preparation is also made as a side product from this urine and is used for slimming cures.

Below are two examples of the results of scientific research on urine substances which have a proven curative effect in the case of cancer. The discovery of these kind of substances in urine helps to bring onto a more scientific level the understanding of the positive effects of urine therapy in treating cancer.

– In the 1960s the Nobel Prize winner Albert Szent-Gyorgi (who also discovered vitamin C) isolated a substance in urine called *3-methyl glyoxal*. It has subsequently been proven that this substance destroys cancer cells.

– A certain Dr. S. Burzynski isolated a peptide component in human urine called *Antineoplaston*. It is now known that this substance selectively combats the growth of cancer cells without fighting the growth of normal cells. (see also the letter of Dr. Burzynski to the urine therapy centre in Ahmedabad, India, in Chapter 6).

Many substances with an anti-cancer effect have since been discovered in urine, a number of which are listed and briefly discussed in Chapter 5. It has been discovered that the substance laetrile (also referred to as vitamin B17) is extremely effective in the treatment of cancer. Although it was initially not known how this substance could be produced, it was subsequently discovered that when goats were fed almonds and apricot pips, they produced a usable dose of laetrile in their urine. The following fragment states that human beings are also considered capable of producing such doses of laetrile:

"Also we as human beings produce a small amount of laetrile when consuming apricots pips and (almond pits). For thousands of years, in very old traditions of medicine, cancer patients have been treated with urine. For us it might be interesting to see what happens when we would replace salted and roasted peanuts, not at all a healthy source of nutrition, with the pips from almonds and apricots."
(From: *Pleidooi voor Biologische Kankerbestrijding,*
P.H.W.A.M. van de Veer, p. 60.)

A short time ago it was discovered that fetuses in the womb use their amniotic fluid in order to develop their lungs. The fetus literally 'breathes' this fluid into its lungs, and without this fluid the lungs cannot develop properly. The fetus's urine is the most important component of amniotic fluid. It has also been discovered that surgery carried out in the womb does not leave a scar. The amniotic fluid, and specifically the urea in it, in which the fetus floats ensures a perfect healing of every wound within the womb.

In the book *The Heart of Healing*, the author William Poole describes how remarkably well the scars of fetuses which are operated upon are healed: as if nothing had happened, whereas, after birth, the same operations would have left big scars that would never completely disappear. Doctors were very surprised to discover this and, according to Poole, they are trying to

find out the reason behind it as they are looking for a method to help heal post-operative scars on adults. Hopefully, some time in the future, they will discover the very simple method of using the patients urine for this purpose! People who are familiar with urine ther-

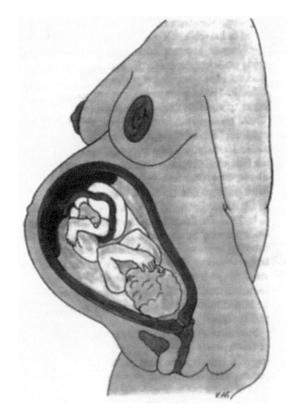

Urine therapy before we are born? A fetus floats in amniotic fluid, which consists mainly of urine. The fetus drinks some of this fluid every day, and urinates it out again: a cycle which helps build up the body and internal organs.

apy know from their own experience how extremely effective just a cloth soaked in urine and placed on a wound can be in healing this wound.

In spite of all these data, the medical world has not as yet taken the step forward to research urine and its effects as a complete entity, even though the beneficial use of many of the components of urine is already acknowledged and exploited.

For example 'Enzymes of America', an American company, has developed a special filter which collects the proteins found in male urine in the 10,000 portable toilets owned by its subsidiary firm, Porta-John. Urine contains small amounts of proteins produced by the body, a number of which are medically very important, such as growth hormones and insulin. There is an annual market of 500 million dollars for these types of substances, which are usually produced by extremely complicated and expensive methods, such as cell cloning. The company is working on bringing its first important product, Urokinase, on the market. Urokinase is an enzyme which dissolves blood clots and is used in treating heart attack victims. The company has contracts for supplying this enzyme to several prominent pharmaceutical companies.

This method was more or less copied from the Chinese. In Shanghai, urine is collected in large basins in the public toilets. The city government then sells the urine to the pharmaceutical companies who extract Urokinase, among other things, from this urine. This is exported and sold as medicine all over the world.

2.4   Recent Research, Practice and Literature

In the past few years, some people from within the medical world have shown an increased interest in urine therapy, particularly doctors who specialize in natural medicine and its principles.

In 1991, Dr. Johann Abele wrote a revised version of the book previously written by Dr. Herz, published under the same title (*Die Eigenharn-behandlung: nach Dr. med. Kurt Herz; Erfahrungen und Beobachtungen*). Abele's book, however, contains only part of the preface from the original book and discusses in a scientific manner the various applications of urine therapy, particularly in the form of urine injections. Dr. Abele realizes that there is no scientific proof for the effects of urine therapy, but still seriously recommends this therapy to the medical world:

> *"Although a lot of research in the field of Auto-Urine therapy was done before the Second World War and well known researchers were reported*

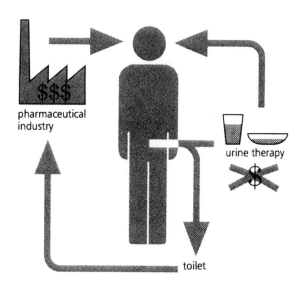

Urine therapy and the pharmaceutical industry: two different cycles.

to have excellent results with it, it will surprise any unbiased observer that after 1945 this therapy – like many other empirical systems of natural medicine – disappeared and was no longer openly subject to research and discussion. It has since only been preserved and developed by those who work outside the field of orthodox medicine.

During this modern era when pure physics and mathematics have entered into areas where science and religion – once strong enemies – can meet each other, it can no longer be tolerated that people dismiss such an interesting method of folk medicine by just saying that it must be a remain of the magical, dirt practice used by uncivilized tribes. An ineffective therapy does not survive hundreds of years in the consciousness of people! The astounding results which therapists who work with this auto-urine-method have over and over again should bring them as well as others to use this therapy for otherwise 'incurable diseases', even though so far no explanation for its effectiveness has been given. For the most important task of a doctor should be, even when in opposition to public opinion and customs, to use any therapy which promises results, in accordance with an old saying: WHO HEALS, IS RIGHT."

(From: *Die Eigenharnbehandlung: nach Dr. med. Kurt Herz; Erfahrungen und Beobachtungen*, Dr. med. Johann Abele, 8., verbesserte Auflage, Karl F. Haug Verlag, Heidelberg, 1991, p. 71-72.)

Besides the previously mentioned book by Carmen Thomas, another book was published in 1993 in Germany on urine therapy entitled *Die Heilkraft der Eigenharntherapie* ('The Healing Power of Urine Therapy'), written by Ingeborg Allmann, a former pharmacist. As with many other people who started to work with urine therapy, it was a personal health crisis which brought her into contact with this method of healing. Ingeborg Allmann suffered from severe allergic asthma, and allopathic medicine offered little relief. After some time, she developed an aversion to all chemical products, the former source of her income. In a complete turnaround, she turned to natural medicine, including urine therapy. Ultimately, Allmann wrote a book about her experiences in which she discusses urine therapy as well as a number of general principles of holistic therapies.

"More than any other method, urine therapy represents the principles of natural medicine, according to which one should not passively depend on 'being healed', but should instead heal oneself actively.

One's own urine is a specific medicine for anyone who is ill – it is made for him or her personally and is just right for what he or she needs at the present moment – because it changes its composition all the time.

It is not only something that cures, but it also sustains health when taken as a preventative.

Taken energetically, one could consider urine to be an exact hologram of both healthy as well as diseased body fluids. All information from the body fluids is collected and stored in the urine.

Since everyone has to learn to take responsibility for their own health over and over again – do you normally give your highest good so easily in the hands of others? – anyway, urine therapy will help you in a very simple way to take that responsibility with your own hands."

(From: *Die Heilkraft der Eigenharn-Therapie*, Ingeborg Allmann, Verlag Dr. Karl Höhn KG, Biberach 1993, p. 5-6.)

Allmann emphasizes the importance of fasting, particularly during chronic illnesses. She also explains how urine can be injected, and describes another method in which urine and blood are mixed. A few drops of this mixture should then be ingested orally on a regular basis. This shows the versatility of the different methods of application of urine therapy, although, according to Allmann, drinking, and specifically fasting, is the most simple and effective way.

Allmann discusses the kidneys as a source of primal energy which is essential for the body. The kidneys are vital organs which play an extremely important role in the balance of the whole organism and the functioning of other organs. According to Allmann, urine therapy is an excellent way to restore and stimulate this primal energy.

"Since one's own urine is the best medicine for the kidneys that we could imagine, all diseases which are caused by under- or non-functioning of this organ can be cured in this way, i.e. via the kidneys.

It is clear for any holistic health practitioner that all cycles within the body are interconnected, and this means that the healing of one of those cycles will have a positive effect on the others."

(From: *Die Heilkraft der Eigenharn-Therapie*, Ingeborg Allmann, Verlag Dr. Karl Höhn KG, Biberach 1993, p. 24.)

Allmann extensively describes the role of the pH-value and how important the acid-alkaline percentage is for our body and health. She also gives an overview of the diversity of illnesses on which urine therapy has had positive results. Both Allmann and Abele state that candidiasis (a frequently occurring, stubborn fungal infection) can be completely cured by a three-week urine fast.

Allmann (a pharmacist) also outlines the chemical composition of urine.

In his book *Die Apotheke in uns; Behandlung mit Eigenharn – eine bewährte Naturheilmethode* ('The Pharmacy Within Ourselves; Treatment with Auto-Urine – A Proven Natural Healing Method'), the Swiss physician, Dr. U.E. Hasler, discusses the substances found in urine even more extensively. Hasler tells how, shortly after World War II, he first heard of urine therapy. Urine was often used at the front, for lack of other medication and as a disinfectant for surgery instruments. His interest was rekindled much later when he heard the story of a doctor from Russia. Apparently, this doctor treated many people from far and wide, and was able to alleviate or completely cure illnesses with nothing else than urine therapy, while other methods up until then had failed.

Hasler wanted to know more about urine therapy, and asked Mantak Chia, an Eastern teacher in the field of holistic health and spirituality who is also well-known in the West, for more information:

"I went to the teacher of the course, Mantak Chia, and asked him if he had ever heard of this peculiar method. Immediately his face turned into a big smile, and he pointed at himself and said: "I use it myself. You Western doctors make a big mistake in thinking that the kidneys only discard poisonous substances. Just look at the dung of plants. A human being is also such a plant and can benefit enormously from it.""

(From: *Die Apotheke in uns; Behandlung mit Eigenharn – eine bewährte Naturheilmethode*, Dr. med. U.E. Hasler, Karl F. Haug Verlag, Heidelberg 1994, p.9.)

Hasler ascribes the effect of urine therapy in part to the many effective substances found in urine. He illustrates this with an overview of these substances (almost twenty pages!) and their possible effects. But

Hasler does not limit himself to the medical aspects of these substances; he also discusses the 'life energy' found in urine:

"Looking at the surprising diversity of substances found in urine makes us understand its positive effect. A-L (auto-liquidum=urine, tr.) represents a living substance. This fluid is full of life and contains the life energy which is so important.

In complementary medicine we already deal with the principle of life energy. We have inside our human bodies an inner healing principle; it is what I call "the Healer Within". This inner doctor is very intelligent and wants to keep the organism healthy whenever possible – whether it is a plant, animal or human being. Independently and from within areas we are normally not aware of, he is always busy, never sleeps, does not know Sundays nor holidays, and is always there as long as the organism is alive."

(From: *Die Apotheke in uns; Behandlung mit Eigenharn – eine bewährte Naturheilmethode*, Dr. med. U.E. Hasler, Karl F. Haug Verlag, Heidelberg 1994, p. 48.)

A few brief examples of the use of urine therapy in a number of other countries follow below.

Various schools and clinics in the United States which work with natural medicine also work with urine therapy. The Water of Life Institute in Florida (now Lifestyle Institute, Ruidoso NM) has contributed much to the promotion of the therapy. In New York City, a support group currently exists for those who use urine therapy, with some 700 members, many of whom are suffering from AIDS. Recently I heard about a similar support group existing in West Hollywood, California. Some people with AIDS have already benefited greatly from this therapy.

In 1994 the book *Your Own Perfect Medicine*, written by Martha Christy, was published in the United States. This book gives a very complete and good overview of scientific material concerning the medical value of urine and its substances.

Urine therapy is also used extensively in an institute in England. This institute is directed by Arthur Lincoln Pauls, a specialist in bio-orthonomy and author of the book on urine therapy, *Shivambu Kalpa*. A 'juicier' example of the use of urine therapy in England is the British actress Sarah Miles. She drinks a glass of her own life water daily and swears that this keeps her healthy and beautiful. Urine is terrific for skin care, a fact already well known by the ancient Egyptians. The present-day cosmetic industry is also aware of this fact: if you study the ingredients of a number of skin creams and various brands of toothpaste, you will regularly come across 'urea' as a significant component.

Two books have recently been published in France on urine therapy. The book *Amaroli* suggests a list of names for urine therapy, including the playful name 'pipi-thérapie'. Besides an extensive summary of its practical application, *Amaroli* also places urine therapy within the broader perspective of modern holistic medicine and health concepts. One chapter discusses the transformative and (self)-regenerative effect of drinking urine. From this perspective, urine therapy is a modern way of 'sanctifying' the body, as it revitalizes the genetic structure on the deepest level. We see here a link to the 'sacred' character of urine therapy as described by ancient traditions.

As a conclusion to this section, I would like to focus on a number of facts related to drinking urine in emergency situations.

Drinking urine is a good alternative wherever water is scarce. It not only satisfies the need for liquid, but also actually keeps the body healthy. Some time ago there was an earthquake in Egypt. A survivor was pulled out of the rubble in Cairo after being trapped for three days. The man had kept himself alive by, among other things, drinking his own urine and he was in excellent condition. I heard another story about a man who kept himself alive with his own urine for a week in a collapsed mine. At the time of his rescue, he looked fine and was in extraordinary health. I also recently read an article about an Italian athlete who was lost in the Sahara for ten days. Upon returning to the civilized world, he told how he had drunk his own urine for lack of other liquids. He had kept himself alive by eating desert plants and insects and drinking his own urine.

Shipwrecked people can drink their own urine to survive, although one should not wait until the body is almost dehydrated before doing so. Drinking urine is also a smart way to survive in situations in which water is unsafe to drink. During earthquakes and floods, water is often infected with pathogens, while urine is always sterile. Drinking polluted water can cause serious, often fatal, illnesses. Urine is a perfect alternative: if drunk fresh, it quenches thirst without presenting any danger, and is always available – any time, anywhere. Moreover, it will help combat possible diseases.

Soldiers have survived long periods in the wilderness by drinking their own urine, and soldiers in the Foreign Legion are sometimes instructed to rub their own urine into their skin in order to build up resistance to illness. Soldiers sometimes also urinate into their shoes before starting on a march, as urine apparently helps prevent blisters. The method of using urine for (new) shoes was often applied in the past and even today I sometimes meet people from the older generation who still know how to get their shoes fitting by using this versatile fluid.

3. NECTAR OF IMMORTALITY:
The History of Urine Therapy in the East

3.1 Urine Therapy within Hinduistic Tradition

Urine therapy is associated with Ayurveda, sometimes referred to as 'mother of all medicine.' Ayurveda is an ancient form of naturopathy and is still being applied and practiced in India. Presently, it is becoming more popular in the West as well. In India, a 5,000-year-old document has been found which describes the practice of urine therapy. In this document, there are many references to herbs and medicines still used in present day Ayurveda.

This document consists of 107 verses (slokas), is called *Shivambu Kalpa Vidhi* ('the method of drinking urine in order to rejuvenate'), and is part of a document called *Damar Tantra*. (The entire text can be found in Chapter 7.)

Shivambu literally means the water of Shiva, the highest god in the Indian pantheon. The name Shiva means *auspiciousness*. In India, at least among urine therapists, one often speaks of drinking Shivambu, which simply means drinking the water of auspiciousness.

These are the opening verses of the *Damar Tantra* text, in which the god Shiva begins to speak with his wife Parvati:

Verses 1–4
"Oh Parvati! (The God Shiva speaks to his wife Parvati.) Those who practice this method can enjoy the fruits of their meditation and this method. For this, certain actions have been recommended along with certain types of utensils. The Shivambu is to be drunk from pots made of gold, silver, copper, brass, iron, tin, glass, earth, bamboo, bones, leather, or a bowl made of plantain leaves.

The urine should be collected in any one of the above mentioned utensils and should be drunk. However, earthen pots are the best for use."

Practical instructions are given on how to collect and ingest urine, and advice on what is best to eat if you drink your own urine. It has to be kept in mind, however, that this document was written for those who practice yoga, work intensively with their body and soul and adapt their food to this lifestyle. Nevertheless, the following verse contains some helpful general guidelines for everyone who uses urine therapy.

Verse 5
"The follower of the therapy should avoid pungent, salty ingredients in his meals. He should not over-exert himself. He should follow a balanced and light diet..."

Urine was equated with a divine drink which had the power to exterminate all kinds of illnesses and ailments. The following verse suggests that physical purification is connected with a life of meditation.

Verse 9

"Shivambu is a divine nectar! It is capable of abolishing old age and various types of diseases and ailments. The follower should first ingest his urine and then start his meditation."

A number of verses discuss the importance of massaging with urine. This is an important and supplementary part of applying urine therapy, the effects of which will comprehensively be discussed elsewhere in this book. A few verses on massaging with urine follow below.

Verse 44

"Now, oh Parvati, I shall tell you about the process of massage.

If such a massage is carried out, the follower can enjoy the fruits of his meditation and his lifestyle and will experience spiritual growth."

तस्य मन्त्रं प्रवक्ष्यामि ग्रहणादानसर्जने ।
मंत्र: ॥ ॐ ह्रीं क्लीं भैरवाय नम: ॥
अनेन ग्रहणं कुर्याद्योगी यत्नाच्छिवाम्बुन: ।
मंत्र: ॥ ॐ श्रीं क्लीं उड्डामरेश्वराय नम: ॥
अनेनादाय तत्पानं योगी कुर्वन्दोषभाक् ॥४६॥
मंत्र: ॥ ॐ सर्वसृष्टिप्रभवे रुद्राय नम: ॥
अनेन देवि मन्त्रेण प्रयत्नोत्सर्जनं चरेत् ॥४७॥

Part of a Sanskrit text from the Shivambu Kalpa Vidhi *as described in the Damar Tantra.*

Verse 48

"Shivambu should be applied to the whole body. It is exceptionally nourishing, and can relieve all ailments."

Verse 87

"Oh Parvati! If he massages his body thrice a day and night with Shivambu, his countenance will be shining and his heart will be strong. His body and muscles will be strong. He will float in pleasure."

This text is special because it connects physical purification with purity of spirit and state of mind. Verse 87 is an especially good example of this belief. The hormonal component seems to have a positive effect on the state of mind (see Chapter 5). Various people with whom I have spoken felt noticeably more emotionally stable, high-spirited and vital after they started urine therapy.

The last verse of the text, in which Parvati is requested to keep the entire story a secret, follows below:

Verse 107

"Oh my beloved Parvati! I have narrated the details of Shivambu Kalpa. This is its technique. Attempts should be made to keep it a secret. Do not tell anyone."

With this intriguing warning, the chapter on *Shivambu Kalpa Vidhi* as described in the *Damar Tantra* concludes. Another story which I know of by word of mouth is about Shiva telling his wife Parvati how good urine therapy is for physical and spiritual health. A number of incidents occur, however, before Shiva is pressed to divulge the secret to Parvati in this rather juicy story.

The story goes as follows: Shiva and Parvati are happily married, but over the years friction has begun to develop between the two. How has this come about? Parvati is jealous of Shiva because he always looks so handsome and healthy, is extremely vital and has such a zest for life. Furthermore, he maintains that he is immortal. However, whenever Parvati asks Shiva how this is possible, he always answers that it is a secret. Parvati is not satisfied with this answer, and she begins to pressure her husband. She neglects the housekeeping, and when that does not help she burns their meals more and more often. But that does not help either. She finally takes drastic measures: she denies her husband any sexual contact. However, the world and the universe existed by the grace of the sexual intercourse the mighty god Shiva regularly had with his wife Parvati. Heaven and earth shook during their intercourse, and so all life remained in existence. Shiva was faced with a difficult dilemma. He either divulged his secret or the world would come to an end. Ultimately, he decided to tell his secret: the source of his immortality and unbridled vitality was nothing other than drinking his own urine. Parvati now knew the secret, but Shiva warned her to treat this valuable information with respect and not to tell it to just anybody.

Information on urine therapy has survived partly because it is often passed down in secret traditions, one of which is Tantric Yoga. Urine therapy is also called Amaroli in the Tantric Yoga tradition. Amaroli comes from the word *Amar*, which means immortality. Amaroli is used together with certain yoga exercises (Kriya Yoga) to purify the body so that the consciousness can ultimately contain the entire universe. In this respect, it is closely related to a religious practice, and is therefore not really a method of treatment.

Swami Satyananda Saraswati states in *'Amaroli – The Way of the Yogi'*, the preface to the book *Amaroli*:

"I am fully acquainted with the topic of amaroli and have had personal experience with its use. Of course, I did not use it for therapy but in

order to perfect vajroli kriya, and I am convinced that those who want to perfect vajroli will have to go through the process of amaroli.

Since 1943, right up to 1978 (date of publication of the book Amaroli), I have never seen bad results from the use of amaroli, either in therapy or for vajroli. Just recently a very ill gentleman approached me and asked me my opinion on amaroli. I suggested that he try it

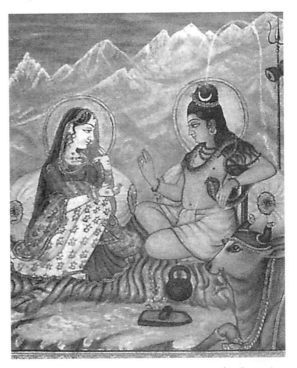

Shiva and his wife Parvati. It was not easy for Parvati to fish the secret out of Shiva, but he ultimately told her. Nonetheless it is information that should be treated carefully, he warns her.

for himself and see what happens. Now, two months later, he has recovered completely.

From the healing point of view, if amaroli proves to be less dangerous than the therapeutic use of drugs, synthetic hormones and various other assorted chemical substances, if it proves less corrosive and nutritionally harmful than Coca Cola and 7-Up, if it is less dependence-producing and intoxicating than alcohol, less distasteful than eating gelatin, manufactured from the hooves and tendons of animals, then I am sure it will be a boon to humanity.

I personally feel that we must state the facts on amaroli in as straightforward, clear and direct a manner as possible. Then mankind may just possibly find that there are many other benefits hidden in the science of amaroli than originally believed."

(From: *Amaroli*, S. S. Saraswati, Bihar School of Yoga, Bihar 1978)

Many verses in the *Damar Tantra* refer to the spiritual aspects of urine therapy. Keep in mind that this text was meant for yogis or monks who followed a spiritual path. A number of things will therefore sound exaggerated. One example is:

Verse 19
"After eight years of working with this method, the follower can conquer all the five important elements of the universe.

Nine years of this method will make the follower immortal."

In the Indian tradition the entire material world consists of the five elements earth, water, fire, air and ether. Conquering these elements is equal to spiritual freedom, which means one does not have to remain in the cycle of reincarnation. Generally stated, reincarnation is based upon the belief that a person keeps being reborn until he is liberated from earthly life, either by performing good deeds or by becoming enlightened.

In this sense reaching immortality can be seen as achieving spiritual freedom.

Other fragments in the *Damar Tantra* refer to the influence of urine therapy on moods and character.

It is also clear that urine therapy is applied in combination with herbs. The method of urine therapy described in the *Damar Tantra* is closely related to the Ayurvedic tradition, Ayurveda being the 'science of long life', an Indian system of natural medicine and living, thousands of years old and still successfully being practiced. The following fragments indicate how urine therapy relates to Ayurveda and to herbs blended according to Ayurvedic principles:

Verse 37
"Sulphur, dried fruit of Amla (Phylonthus Emblica) and nutmeg powder should be mixed together and taken daily, followed by Shivambu. All pains and miseries vanish."

Verse 62
"The follower who drinks the mixture of Shivambu and the powder of the five parts of the Sharapunkha (Devnal) plant will become the master and authority of meditation. He will enjoy utmost pleasure in life."

Verse 85
"Oh Goddess, if in the early morning the follower nasalizes his own urine, the ailments arising out of Kapha, Pitta and Vata will vanish. He will have a healthy appetite and his body will become strong and healthy."

Other ancient texts which are part of the religious and spiritual heritage of India also contain fragments about and refer either to urine therapy or to 'amaroli' ('nectar of immortality'). A number of these fragments, most of them taken over from the book *Amaroli* of S.S. Saraswati, follow below.

Hatha Yoga Pradipika 3;96–97
"In the doctrine of the Kapalikas, amaroli is the drinking of the midstream, leaving the first for it is too pungent (too much bile) and the last, which is useless. He who drinks amari, snuffs it daily, and practises vajroli, is said to be practicing amaroli."

Gyanarnava Tantra, Chapter 22
"After realizing the exact knowledge of dharma and adharma, every aspect of the world becomes holy – stool, urine, ovum, nails, bones, are all holy things in the sight of that person who has explored mantra.

O Parvati, different deities are living in that water from which urine is made, then why is urine said to be contaminated?"

Harit, Chapter 1 on Urine
"Human urine is basic, bitter and light. It destroys diseases of the eyes, makes the body strong, improves digestion and destroys coughs and colds."

Bhawa Prakasha, Verse 7, Chapter on Urine
"Human urine destroys poison, properly used it gives new life, purifies blood, clears skin troubles, is sharp in taste and contains many salts."

Yoga Ratnakar, Mutrashtakam Verse 11
"Human urine controls bile in the blood, destroys worms, cleans intestines, controls cough and calms nerves. It is sharp in taste, destroys laziness and is an antidote to poisons."

Sushrut Samhita, 4/2 28
"Human urine is an antidote to poisons."

Tirumandiram
(written by Siddhar Tirumoolar), Verse 830
"Shivambu is medicine for the courageous. It is divine and nectar, the gift of shakti, and imbues one with great strength. The God Nandi has told us about this. The great sages have said it is the basis of all medicines."

Vyavahar Sutra, Chapter 42
In Chapter 42 of the Vyavahar Sutra, a religious document from the Jain tradition written by Acharya Bhadrabahu, the followers' pratimas (promises and trials) are listed. This includes a period as a hermit during which one fasts and drinks all one's secreted urine.

Shiva-Parvati Sambad
This is an ancient Sanskrit document studied by Professor Athawale from Ahmedabad. The text was apparently terribly damaged, but in spite of this Professor Athawale has been able to decipher the following fragments.

Shiva says to his wife Parvati
"Devi, listen to what I say: Shivambu (urine) is a great purifier; it removes all the impurities from the body. Shivambu is a veritable nectar (amrit) churned out of one's own body."

"The pot which is to be used for collecting urine before oral consumption should first be cleansed with a piece of cloth. While cleaning the pot the following mantra should be uttered – 'astraya phut'."

The text includes the following mantra, which should be said aloud seven times before drinking urine:

"Om, aim hreem amritodbhave amrita varshini, amritam kuru no swaha."

A mantra is a holy saying which can be compared to a short prayer. The super mantras *Om Namaha Shivaya* ('All honor to Shiva' or 'May Thy will be done') from Hinduism and *Om Manipadme Hum* ('The jewel in the lotus') from Buddhism are also known to many Westerners.

The text further states that for fast results, urine should be drunk three times a day: once in the morning, once in the afternoon and once in the evening, usually one hour before or after dinner. One of the results of this can be:

"By taking shivambu continually and regularly, a man or woman becomes sexually potent and the signs of old age (such as senility and loss of procreative power) are removed."

Satapatha Brahmana
"The Soma (moon) beverage is urine."

The Vedic tradition links the use of hallucinogenic substances and the drinking of urine. Soma was a drink brewed from hallucinogenic plants. Which plant that was is still unknown, although many suggestions have been made. The following is stated in the above mentioned book *Plants of the Gods*:

"The Rig-Veda definitely refers to urine-drinking in the Soma ritual: "The swollen men piss the flowing Soma. The lords, with full bladders, piss Soma quick with movement." The priests impersonating Indra and Vayu, having drunk Soma in milk, urinate Soma. In the Vedic poems, urine is not offensive but is an ennobling metaphor to describe rain: the blessings of rain are likened to showers of urine, and the clouds fertilize the earth with their urine."

(From: *Plants of the Gods; Their Sacred Healing and Hallucinogenic Powers*, Evans Schultes, R. & Hofmann, A., Healing Arts Press, Rochester Vermont 1992, p. 83.)

Urine therapy is still used today by yogis within the

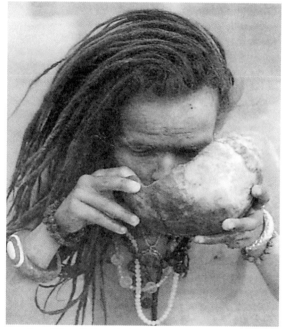

A saddhu (Indian holy man) drinking urine from a human skull. Australian scientists are doing research into the drinking of urine by Indian yogis and the presumed beneficial effects on their meditation practices. The tranquillizing effects of morning urine are, according to the hypothesis of the scientists, to be attributed to a hormone called melatonin.

Hindu tradition. The influence of Western morality concerning the body and healing has in this century caused the virtual disappearance of the use of urine by ordinary people in India, who nowadays often place more trust in prescriptions from an allopathic doctor. However, urine therapy has become much more popular since there have been a number of books written on the subject and published in several Indian languages.

Initially Dr. Armstrong's book caused renewed interest in urine therapy. Soon afterwards, a book was published by Raojibhai Patel, who has since re-popularized urine therapy in India. Patel was a well-known freedom fighter and assistant to Mahatma Ghandi. He applied the therapy to himself and fully recovered from asthma and a heart condition. As a result, he wrote *Manav Mootra* in 1959, a highly informative book translated into at least three languages and of which more than 100,000 copies have been sold.

The practical application of urine therapy has since then gained much ground in India. There are even a few clinics where people can be treated with urine therapy. The therapy is also used successfully in a Christian hospital, the Bethany Colony, where leprosy patients are treated. Leprosy is said to be brought fully into remission by adding small amounts of the patient's urine to a glass of orange juice each morning.

Making this free and effective method of treatment available for many people seems very important in a poor country such as India. The former prime minister of India, Morarji Desai, has contributed greatly to this, so that nowadays an estimated 30.000 people in Bombay alone and 300.000 people in the Indian state of Gujarat practice urine therapy!

It is interesting to note that according to Armstrong many people in India unknowingly enjoyed the blessings of urine therapy by simply bathing in the Ganges, although, with the increase in pollution in India this is less likely to be the case. Armstrong:

"Those who read that widely known book Mother India *may remember some passages therein devoted to the 'filthy habits' of the native peoples. Among the health 'superstitions' its authoress pointed out, was the belief that the waters of one part of a famous river in North Middle India possesses healing properties. People bathed in and drank its waters.*

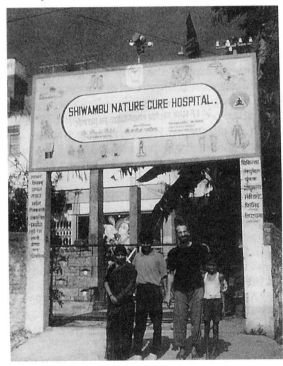

A clinic where urine therapy is practiced in Kolhapur, India. Written above the entrance: Shivambu Nature Cure Hospital. In India urine therapy is often called Shivambu, the water of Shiva.

Wondering whether there could be something more than faith in the cures effected, she had samples of the water analyzed by European analysts. The healing liquid proved to be nothing more than a weak solution of urine and aqua pura!"

(From: *The Water of Life*, J.W. Armstrong, Health Science Press, London 1971, p. 125.)

In India, drinking cow urine is a commonly accepted practice, as a preventive measure and in the treatment of malaria. A number of Westerners I met in India also drink cow urine to avoid taking malaria tablets daily for months on end. I do not take anti-malaria tablets either while I travel in India, but simply trust the effects of drinking my own life water.

One of the urine therapists whom I met in India told me that cow urine contains an enormous lot of enzymes which support and stimulate an optimal functioning especially of the liver. This helps the body to cope with a possible diseased condition, even in the case of serious illnesses such as malaria. He told me that for that reason he also half jokingly advises his patients to eat like a cow when applying urine therapy in an intensive form in case of a serious illness. The serious undertone of this advice is, of course, that a mainly raw-food, vegetarian diet enhances the healing effects of one's own human urine used for drinking.

I found the following quotation on the use of cow urine by a certain Abbé Dubois in *Mother India*:

"'Urine is looked upon as the most efficacious for purifying any kind of uncleanness. I have often seen... Hindus following the cows to pasture, waiting for the moment when they could collect the precious liquid in vessels of

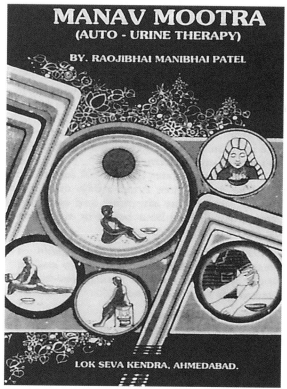

Urine bestseller in India:
Manav Mootra *(Human Urine)*.

brass, and carrying it away while still warm to their houses. I have also seen them waiting to catch it in the hollow of their hands, drinking some of it and rubbing their faces and heads with the rest. Rubbing it in this way is supposed to wash away all external uncleanness, and drinking it, to cleanse all internal impurity.'
Very holy men, adds the Abbé, drink it daily."

(From: *Mother India*, Katherine Mayo, Harcourt, Brace and Co., New York 1927, p.225)

3.2　Medical Use of Urine within Buddhist Tradition

References to urine therapy can also be found in the Buddhist and Taoist traditions. Buddha himself had a thorough knowledge of Ayurveda and was aware of the power of urine therapy. In the Buddhist document, *Mahabagga*, it is said that Buddha advised the use of urine in case of poison by a snake bite.

Milarepa, the great Tibetan Buddhist yogi saint, once said:

"At times when I am thirsty, I drink pure blue water.
At others I rely on my own secretions.
Frequently I drink the flow from the Fountain of Compassion.
Quite often I sip enchanting nectar of goddesses."

Urine therapy was possibly spread throughout Tibet, Mongolia and China along with Buddhism. Many lamas (Tibetan monks) easily attained the age of one hundred with the help of urine. One of the well-known climbers of Mount Everest, Sir Morris Wilson, had also heard about the use of urine from the lamas. He practiced urine therapy during his expeditions by drinking urine as well as massaging it into his skin. He was therefore able to withstand all the rigors of the difficult trek.

I came across a number of Tibetan monks a few years ago while waiting for my plane back to Amsterdam at the airport in New Delhi. With the help of an interpreter, I asked them if they knew about urine therapy. They proceeded to tell me that although they did not usually drink their own urine, they did drink the urine of one of the higher lamas if one of the monks fell ill. They believe that urine from one of the higher lamas is purer and cleaner. Purity of mind is always connected with physical purity in the Eastern tradition. I spoke with people in India who practiced an intensive Vipassana meditation and simultaneously applied urine therapy. They noticed that over the course of the ten-day Vipassana meditation their urine became clearer and purer. Research on acid-alkaline proportions has demonstrated that stress causes the blood and therefore the urine to acidify. Reduction or prevention of stress, brought about by meditation, naturally improves the quality of the blood.

Tibetan medicine sometimes prescribes urine therapy for the mentally ill, and includes an ancient

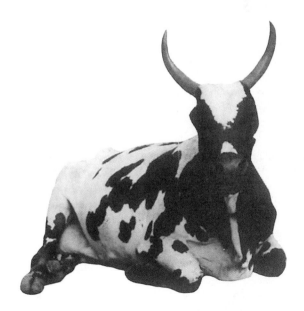

The cow is a holy animal in India. Apart from this belief, cow urine has proved to be a fantastic medicine for various illnesses and ailments.

tradition in which urine is used for diagnosing physical as well as mental symptoms, varying from simple (physical) ailments to possession by demons and spirits.

In her book *Tibetan Buddhist Medicine and Psychiatry*, Terry Clifford refers to the use of urine in a number of prescriptions. These prescriptions are found in the *Gyu-zhi*, the most important medical document in Tibetan medical literature. Clifford believes that the use of urine is one of the many influences of Ayurveda on Tibetan medicine: *"Urine was extensively used as medication in Ayurveda medicine, especially for the mentally ill."*

The following are two prescriptions in which reference is made to the use of urine:

Gyu-zhi, from Chapter 77
(on exorcising spirits)

"All these elemental spirits are swiftly liberated by the use of an edible ointment and snuff called "medicine butter." It is compounded of:
the three chief fruits [Chebulic myrobalan-arura, Beleric myrobalan, Emblic myrobalan], sandal-wood, saffron crocus, bya-kri, the three hots [ginger, long pepper, black pepper], cardamom, barberry, pine, Fanacetum sibiricum, Holarrhena anti-dysenterica, pu-shel-rtsi [khus-khus or orchid], white mustard, Indian valerian, juniper, lavender, Piper chaba, Costus speciosus, hellebore, white aconite, spang-ma, realgar, the "six urines"."

(From: *Tibetan Buddhist Medicine and Psychiatry*, Terry Clifford, Samuel Weiser Inc., York Beach USA 1984, p. 181-182.)

Gyu-zhi, from Chapter 78
"For disturbance from poison, rely upon a tablet made of:
dpa-ser, white aconite, red aconite, re-ral, turmeric, "fragrant water" [urine]."

(From: *Tibetan Buddhist Medicine and Psychiatry*, Terry Clifford, Samuel Weiser Inc., York Beach USA 1984, p. 188.)

In an accompanying note this is further explained:
"Mix the powder of the above with red cow's urine. The cow must have been inside a house for seven days and should have had clean grass to eat. The urine should be taken at sunrise, then strained and then boiled with the powder until it yields a thick paste. Urine, especially that of a healthy and clean person or animal, is believed to be an excellent antiseptic and anti-toxin. It can be applied directly to an open wound to prevent infection if nothing else is available. Here it is used to counter an internal toxic reaction."

(From: *Tibetan Buddhist Medicine and Psychiatry*, Terry Clifford, Samuel Weiser Inc., York Beach USA 1984, p. 190-191.)

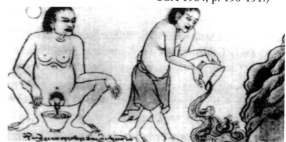

Partial representation of a Tibetan Thangka, which 'demonstrates' how one may diagnose illnesses by examining (looking at) someone's urine.

Clifford writes the following on the use of urine in Ayurveda and Tibetan medicine in general:

"As for the inclusion of substances such as blood and urine in medicines, it may strike the modern mind as disgusting and outrageous. But such substances are found in traditional medicines around the world, including China, and sometimes turn out, under scientific investigation, to have some merit. Urine, for example, has recently been found to contain substances that act as powerful mental and emotional tranquilizers without any of the side-effects of manufactured chemical tranquilizers – according to Danish scientists."
(From: *Tibetan Buddhist Medicine and Psychiatry*,
Terry Clifford, Samuel Weiser Inc., York Beach
USA 1984, p. 209.)

Tibetan doctors who visit the West even today can make extremely precise diagnoses based upon a single glance at a fresh glass of the patient's urine. They also advise those who work with precious stones to urinate on the stones. This protects the stone and makes it entirely the possession of the person who works with it or wears it. A thin layer of body-specific information, as it were, covers the stone.

In his bestseller *Seven Years in Tibet: My Life With the Dalai Lama*, the Austrian mountain climber Heinrich Harrer describes how he was interned in India during World War Two, subsequently fled to Tibet and after numerous adventures befriended and became the teacher of the Dalai Lama. During his travels throughout Tibet, he learned the Tibetan customs and traditions, and heard about the use of urine as medicine. As a 'normal' Westerner, Harrer was quite skeptical about this method:

"All things which had served for the personal use of the Dalai Lama were regarded as the best remedies against illness or charms against evil spirits. People used to compete for the cakes and fruits which I used to bring home with me from His Holiness's kitchen, and I could not give my friends greater pleasure than by sharing these things with them. They would eat them immediately and were convinced that there wasn't anything which would protect them better than these.

But that was still relatively harmless. I had much less understanding for the fact that people would drink the urine of the living Buddha – something which was wanted most of all but nevertheless only rarely given out. The Dalai Lama himself would only shake his head and he did not like it when someone asked for it. But he alone was not able to go against all these customs and consequently he did not bother too much about it. And then again, in India one could always see people in the streets drinking the urine of holy cows."
(From: *Sieben Jahre Tibet: Mein Leben am Hofe des Dalai Lama*, Heinrich Harrer, Ullstein,
Frankfurt/M-Berlin, p. 387, author's translation)

"We found that the people had more confidence in the laying-on of hands and faith-healing than in the ministration of the monks of the schools of medicine. The Lamas often smear their patients with their holy spittle. Tsampa, butter and the urine of some saintly man are made into a sort of gruel and administered to the sick."
(From: *Seven Years in Tibet*, Heinrich Harrer,
Granada, London 1984)

Nowadays urine therapy is promoted in Taiwan by a Urine therapy Hotline. According to a newspaper article I received from India, some 200,000 Taiwanese drink their own urine daily.

The monks in a Buddhist monastery in the north of Taiwan also promote urine therapy. The twenty monks and approximately 2,000 followers at this monastery faithfully practice urine therapy. Furthermore, they distribute brochures in Buddhist bookstores and restaurants. Another Buddhist in Taiwan recently published a book (not yet translated) entitled, 'The Magic Golden Water Cure', a collection of stories of people who were seriously ill and who recovered by drinking urine.

Urine therapy is also being used on an increasingly wider scale in Korea and Japan. In Japan, more than two million people use urine therapy. I recently got hold of a Japanese book on urine therapy of which the title (in translation) reads *'Information Water': The Memory of Water Containing Enormous Healing Power*.

In his book *Cancer Cures In Twelve Ways*, A.A. Cordero discusses the alleged positive effects of urine therapy in the treatment of cancer. Cordero, from the Philippines, refers to the following comments from a Swedish doctor practicing traditional medicine. As the conclusion to this chapter, this serves as an excellent illustration of the interaction between the history of urine therapy in the West and in the East:

"In explaining the virtues of urine in health, Dr. Karl A.B. Helm Y Strand from Europe explained: "Your God Father in Heaven as Creator had given you at your time of birth to this green earth a very precious birth gift in the form of two royal medical factories and these are your own two kidneys. These kidneys produce just for you and not for anyone else the best medicine at any moment in your life for any disease which can hit you. And if you are clever enough to receive the gift of these two royal factories then your body benefits. Don't forget to take advantage of your own birth gift of your precious machine. When you feel you are going to be sick or when already sick drink it every day, morning, noon and afternoon. You can always with this drink meet every disease besetting you.

In the beginning before you are fully acquainted to taking your own urine, I recommend you to mix it in a glass half and half with either clear spring water or natural alkaline water. It has a good taste. It is a good drink for your ailments.""

(From: *Cancer Cures in Twelve Ways*, A.A. Cordero, Science of Nature Healing Centre, 1983, p. 400.)

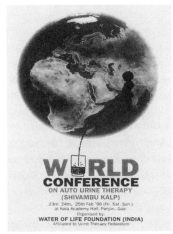

East and West coming together to share their experiences with urine therapy at the World Conference on Auto Urine Therapy in 1996.

4. GOING WITH THE FLOW: The Application of Urine Therapy

4.1 Introductory Remarks

I have discussed the background and history of urine therapy in Chapters 1, 2 and 3; however, the application of urine therapy is ultimately the essence of this book. You can learn the most by practicing it yourself. Since no negative side effects or significant contra-indications have as yet been recorded, everybody can experiment with urine therapy as long as the following conditions are taken into account:

It is generally not recommended to combine urine therapy with the use of (prescribed) chemical, allopathic medicines or recreational drugs. The combination may be dangerous to your health.

If you are taking any form of allopathic medicine, begin with the external application (urine massage) until you are free of all medication, if possible.

If it is not possible or safe to stop the use of certain medicines, start with taking a few drops of urine internally or use a homeopathic tincture. Keep looking and feeling very carefully how you and your body are reacting on the treatment. (See also section *4.5 Warnings and Guidelines*.)

You should also be aware of what you consume while applying urine therapy. Alcohol or coffee consumption or smoking cigarettes can be combined with urine therapy, providing the above mentioned substances are used in moderation. However, the application of urine therapy does not alter the fact that these substances are unhealthy for the human body. The more intensely the therapy is applied, the more precise and aware you should be of what you eat, drink or otherwise use.

Urine therapy can bring about a so-called healing crisis in which the body rapidly detoxifies. This can cause diarrhea, vomiting, rashes, etc. (See also section *4.5 Warnings and Guidelines*.)

Urine therapy consists of two parts: internal application (e.g. drinking urine) and external application (e.g. massaging with urine). Both aspects complement each other and are important for optimal results. The basic principle of urine therapy is therefore quite simple: you drink and massage yourself with urine. Even so, there are a number of different ways to apply urine therapy, the most important of which are discussed below. After your initial experiences, you will be able to determine your own method of application.

As far as the length of any treatment is concerned: be patient and trust the process! Urine therapy helps the body to cleanse and renew itself. Sometimes this takes a lot of time. Urine therapy is as personal as you are. The healing process, its character and its length of time depend upon many factors: the roots of a diseased condition, the intensity with which urine therapy and other methods are applied and, last but not least, your own commitment and faith. With some diseases there are fast results but with chronic diseases it can take weeks, months or even years or a lifetime for the healing process to complete. No matter where your process will lead you or how long it will take, urine therapy will always be helpful to you in some kind of way, if it were only in loving yourself and your body more than you used to.

4.2   The First Sip

Before you decide to drink your first glass of urine, any number of things can pass through your mind. We are all familiar with the taboos surrounding 'pee', which are often more deeply rooted than we think. Even though you may fully acknowledge that drinking urine might be good for your health, perhaps you cannot bring yourself to take that first sip. Do not force yourself into anything; be kind to yourself and give your body and feelings time to adjust to the idea and the practice. While applying urine therapy, listen closely to your body and feelings.

Beatrice Bartnett presents us with some points to think about as far as aversion to urine is concerned: Throughout the civilized world, blood and blood products are used in the medical world without evoking the repugnance associated with urine. We often use prepacked cells, plasma, white blood cells and count-less other blood components. Urine is nothing other than a blood product. We see babies being breast-fed and we are not filled with repugnance. We drink cow's milk and eat cheese from cows, goats and other

animals without a second thought. We eat dairy products in the form of blue cheese (molded) or as sour drinks such as yogurt and buttermilk, not to mention all the other bizarre things which are considered to be delicacies.

Yet we cannot imagine drinking urine. As already discussed, fresh urine simply contains the same sub-stances as those found in blood. What at one moment can be excreted as your urine was part of your blood just minutes before and flowed elsewhere through your body, possibly through your tongue. If it is not poisonous or repugnant while in the blood, why is it suddenly so repulsive as urine?

If it is not the colour (and it is not, because we drink wine, beer and fruit juice of the same colour); and if it is not the smell (and it is not, because we consume considerable amounts of cheese which smell much worse); and if it is not the temperature, then perhaps it is the taste. How many people do you know who have drunk enough urine to really know what it tastes like? Probably not too many. Those who regularly drink their own urine say it tastes mild and not at all unpleasant – a bit salty, like broth or sea water.

A good way to free yourself of this conditioned reaction to the taste is by rinsing or gargling with fresh urine. The taste, the consistency and the feeling will soon become familiar and the repulsion regarding your own rich body fluid will soon be part of the past.

But taking urine into your mouth might be too big a step to begin with. Rubbing a drop into the skin and first smelling your own urine can help you to overcome part of the barrier. Really, it often does not smell bad at all. Many people even like its sometimes sweet odor. More extensive massaging of urine into your skin is also a good way to become accustomed to your own life water.

How can you overcome feelings of aversion to

drinking your own golden elixir? Start by drinking a drop, then a sip each day and slowly build up to a full glass of urine. This is the most comfortable way to allow your body, mind and soul to become accustomed to this therapy.

Another method, which I myself used, is to begin by fasting for a few days. The urine is then so watery that after the second glass you will notice only a slightly salty taste, which makes it much easier to let go of the idea that urine is dirty or at least tastes dirty.

If you still cannot bring yourself to drink your own urine pure, mix a dash of it into a glass of fruit juice or mix it with water and honey. Then try to switch over from the dilution to drinking urine pure.

Once used to that, some people prefer to drink it pure, followed by a glass of water or another healthy liquid. Other people prefer to brush their teeth immediately afterwards.

Once again, make it as easy and pleasant as possible for yourself, especially when beginning urine therapy. Your body and mind deserve patience and love while adjusting to something which up until now might have been considered to be strange or even repulsive. It helps to thank your body before drinking urine in order to acknowledge the value of this golden liquid.

4.3   *Internal Applications*

1. Drinking

Indication: Recommended as a prophylactic; as a rejuvenating tonic; and in minor diseases.

Collect the middle stream of the first morning urine.

The small amounts at the beginning and ending of urination do not have to be collected: the first part rinses the urinary passage clean, so the urine will be as sterile as possible. The last part sometimes contains sediment and is of little value. Only your own, fresh urine should be used.

It is wise to start with a few drops, then a small glass and gradually build up the amount to a level you are comfortable with. This may vary from one to several glasses per day. If you drink your urine not only in the morning but later in the day as well, the urine from approximately one hour after eating is usually the best. Do not eat up to thirty minutes after drinking your urine. After a meal, wait for at least an hour before drinking any urine.

A higher level of hormonal discharge takes place at night when the body completely relaxes and restores itself. Morning urine is therefore the most rich in vital substances.

No extra diet restrictions apply if you drink one glass of morning urine per day, but a diet low in salt and (especially animal) protein is preferable and it will ensure that your urine tastes and smells milder.

However, if you drink urine several times a day, a diet low in protein and salt is essential. A lot of fresh fruit and vegetables are recommended except, of course, when you are fasting on just urine and water, which method will be discussed next. In section *4.6 The Influence of Food*, I will discuss the influence of food and drink on urine.

2. Fasting

Indication: Chronic diseases; cleansing and general fasting. It is important to combine fasting with intensive massage and enemas (see below).

Only your own, fresh urine should be used. You can

fast on urine and water for one or more days; Armstrong sometimes had his patients fast for up to forty-five days. It is advisable to consult a book on fasting before starting, and to conduct longer fasts under trained and, if necessary, medical supervision.

Fasting is in itself a very powerful method of treatment. Urine and water form an extra strong variation and it is best to carry out such a fast step by step.

The following steps are important, especially if you are planning to fast for an extended period of time:

1) *Preparation for the fast*, during which, if necessary, you become accustomed to drinking urine (see *1. Drinking* above). Do not plunge immediately into a full fast, especially if it is your first time!

2) *Before the fast*. Two days before the fast, decrease the intake of protein-rich and heavy foods, especially fried and fatty foods. Fruit and raw vegetables are easily digestible and ensure that the intestines clean themselves so the actual fast can easily begin. In this period, start drinking greater amounts of urine.

3) *The actual fast*. In this period, exclusively drink water and urine. It is best if you do not work during the fast. Although some exertion is possible, rest and relaxation are important in order for the purifying process to take place undisturbed.

In the beginning, stay with drinking the middle stream. Alternated with urine, pure, clean water can be drunk. Once the fast has been in progress for some time, all the urine can be drunk. In this period, you will urinate quite easily: urinating every fifteen minutes is not unusual.

The evening urine may be omitted, so you do not have to get out of bed all the time. A good night's rest is important for the body's recovery process. Evening urine can be saved for other purposes such as massage, compresses, foot baths, etc.

If you start feeling very nauseous, it is advisable to stop the fast. Start the fast again when you feel better.

The length of the actual fast is determined by the type of health problem from which you are suffering. Those who fast for two weeks or more notice that they are rarely hungry. This can be attributed to the alkalinity of urine, which reduces the feeling of hunger, and to the recycling of valuable nutrients such as minerals, hormones and enzymes.

It is not advisable to immediately embark on a prolonged fast, even though such a fast can be very effective. It is definitely more comfortable to start with short urine fasts of one to three days.

During the fast it is important for the person fasting, as well as the assisting (urine-)therapist, to make sure that everything runs smoothly. A healing crisis in the form of diarrhea, vomiting or skin rash is in itself no

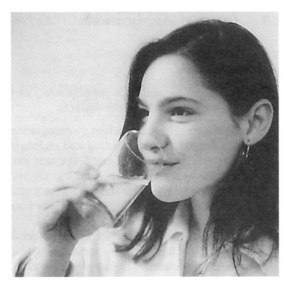

Drinking urine: once you are used to the taste, it's an easy, safe and effective method. You can vary from a few drops up to everything you pass.

cause for worry, but it is advisable to avoid extreme situations. Take your time and fast for a few shorter periods rather than carrying out one long fast which is actually too strenuous.

A complete body massage every day with old, heated urine is highly recommended (see section *4.4 External Applications* for the application and effects of urine massage). Urine massage is good for blood circulation, and massaging with old urine also ensures that you do not have heart palpitations during the fast. Furthermore it serves as a way of feeding the body through the skin, immediately into the muscle and lymph-tissue.

During fasts, urine enemas are highly recommended (see below). Many illnesses begin in the intestines and it is very important to get rid of toxic waste products stored in them and to keep them clean.

4) After the fast. This period is necessary in order to slowly and carefully return to a normal and natural eating pattern. You should take at least one week to gradually and carefully readjust your eating habits. The best way to end a fast is to stop drinking urine and water at the end of the afternoon. After one hour, drink a glass of orange juice, lemon juice with water, grape juice or apple juice. The next day, drink another glass of fruit juice during lunch. From this time on, start eating juicy fruits.

The following day, eat vegetable broth, steamed vegetables and rice. This is a good way to return to your old pattern of eating, excluding the unhealthy habits.

2a. Alternative Fast

Indication: When a total fast is not appropriate or desirable.

If fasting exclusively on water and urine is too great of a strain, consume one light meal per day. This fast proceeds according to the same basic rules as a complete fast, except for a few differences:

1) Eat a light meal consisting of wholemeal bread, brown rice with steamed vegetables, raw vegetables or fruit preferably at the end of the afternoon. Chew the food well.

2) Refrain from eating or drinking (including urine or water) one hour before and after the meal.

This fast can be sustained for quite some time. It is therefore good during illnesses which greatly weaken the body.

3. Enemas

Indication: Small enemas are useful in case of allergies and as a substitute for drinking. Big enemas are recommended for cleansing the intestines, especially when fasting.

The simplest way to administer a small enema is with a syringe containing some urine. You can use fresh or old urine (see section *4.4 External Applications*

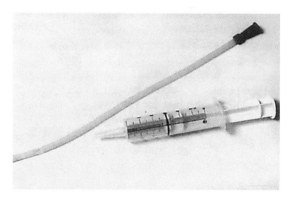

Urine enemas: a good way to clean the bowels and to regenerate its tissues.

regarding old urine). For big enemas the urine can be mixed with warm water. The urine is kept in the intestinal canal as long as possible. There are various ways to administer an enema, and both the amount of liquid and the length of time in which the liquid is kept in the intestines can vary. If you do not know how to administer an enema, it is wise to seek advice or to read up on this.

A number of urine therapists emphasize the importance of enemas, especially with chronic illnesses. During a chronic illness, the body often has a high level of toxicity, which means that poisonous substances can be found in the tissues. Administering an enema is a good way to remove poisonous substances from the body, and especially from the intestines. Furthermore, a number of substances found in urine are better absorbed by the body in this way than by oral ingestion.

4. Gargling

Indication: Throatache; toothache; parodontosis; other ailments of tongue and mouth.

Urine should be kept in the mouth for twenty to thirty minutes or, when that seems too much, as long as possible. Gargling with urine is an effective way to fight gum problems or other mouth and tongue disorders. In addition, toothaches disappear quickly and teeth stay healthy. It can help heal aphts quite fast. After gargling, spit the urine out again.

5. Douching

Indication: Irritation or diseases of vagina and uterus.

A solution of Golden Seal (Hydrastis Canadensis; Canadian Anemone) and urine relieves and heals many vaginal discomforts, and purifies as well. You can also simply wash with fresh or old urine. Douching is recommended for discharge, yeast infections, herpes and tumors.

6. Eye and Eardrops

Indication: Irritation or diseases of the eyes or ears; earaches.

Painful, burning and tired eyes can be relieved by applying a few drops of fresh or boiled urine to the eyes. Eye cups with urine are also quite useful. It is sometimes wise to dilute the urine used for eyedrops with a bit of water.

Eyedrops are very helpful in cases of conjunctivitis. Irritation due to the wearing of contact lenses can disappear or be relieved by this treatment. Regular eye treatments with urine therapy may improve eyesight.

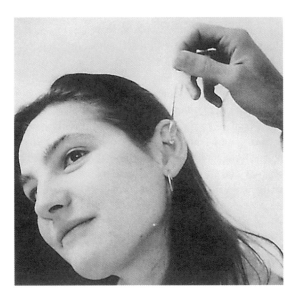

Ear drops with urine.

You can use four-day old urine for earaches or ear infections, as old urine enhances the effect of this method, but fresh urine will do as well. Put some drops in the ears and close them with some cotton wool dipped in oil.

7. Urine sniffing

Indication: Irritation or diseases of the nose, sinuses and eyes.

This method is called Neti within the yoga tradition. Salt water or urine is sniffed in the nose from a small bowl. Sniffing urine is the most effective treatment for a stuffed nose, other sinus disorders such as sinusitis, and problems with the uppermost part of the respiratory canal. This method also affects the eyes positively. If pure urine is too strong, dilute it with water.

Place fresh urine in a cup or dish, if necessary diluted with lukewarm water. Place your nose in this liquid and slowly sniff as much as possible, one nostril at a time. Open your mouth immediately and let the liquid drip out of your mouth. Repeat this a number of times. Blow your nose in order to remove the remaining liquid. You can also use a special Neti-pot for this treatment.

Initially, you may find this method to be unpleasant but you will become accustomed to it after a number of times. If you apply this method regularly, the common cold will soon be a part of the past.

8. Homeopathic tincture

Indication: As a supportive measure; when drinking is not possible or wanted; when healing on subtle levels is required; especially useful when treating allergies.

A 1/1.000.000 solution of urine should be placed under the tongue. Begin with two drops a day and increase this amount to ten drops a day. It is quite easy to prepare this tincture.

a. Purchase a medicine dropper or pipette and six small tubes (available at the chemist or pharmacy).

b. Place eighteen drops of water in each tube and place the tubes in a cup in order to avoid spilling.

c. Collect the middle part of your urine and add two drops of urine to the water in tube 1.

d. Shake the tube 25-50 times. Do this by holding the tube in a closed fist, with your thumb over the opening. Firmly strike your fist in the palm of your other hand. Shaking the tube is very important.

e. Place two drops of liquid from tube 1 in tube 2. Repeat the shaking. Rinse the pipette after each use. Continue the diluting-shaking process until you have reached tube six.

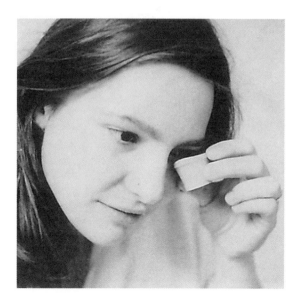

Eye bath with urine.

f. The solution in tube 6 represents a 6∞ or 1/1.000.000 dilution.

This tincture can be applied as often as you wish. Depending on the symptom, the tincture can be applied daily by placing a few drops on the tongue. I myself am not familiar with the practical application of this method. It is particularly useful if you cannot bring yourself to drink urine or if it is not wise to drink urine, e.g. if it contains too much pus.

9. Urine injections

Indication: As a supportive measure; when drinking is not possible or wanted; especially useful when treating allergies.

In Germany, some doctors working with natural

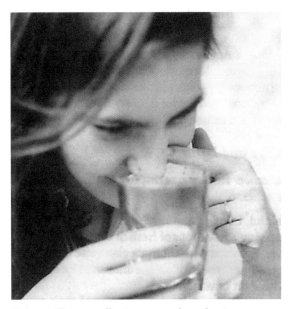

Urine sniffing: an effective way to clean the sinuses.

medicine regularly use this method by injecting urine into the muscles. This method has yielded positive results, particularly in the treatment of various allergies. I myself am not familiar with the practical application of this method. If you wish to inject urine, it is advisable to contact somebody who has experience with this method.

This method is described in more detail in the books by Abele, Hasler and Allmann (see *Bibliography*.)

4.4 External Applications

Urine used for external application works best if it is a few days old and heated. Normally, the urine should be at least four days old, but it can also be kept for a longer period of time. Some people compare it to wine: the longer it ages, the better the fermented final product. I always use urine which is four to eight days old.

It is best to keep urine in a dark brown glass bottle which can be closed with a cork or some cotton wool, or in a bottle or glass pot with the top or lid placed on top of it (rather than screwed on). In this way the bottle or pot is closed while allowing air in, which is necessary for the fermentation process.

The more urine ages, the more alkaline it becomes, as urea decomposes into ammonia. Calcium precipitates during this process, causing old urine to become murky. It is therefore normal for old urine to contain sediment.

The ancient document Shivambu Kalpa Vidhi (see Chapter 7) recommends boiling down urine to one quarter of its volume for use in massage. Practice proves, however, that urine which has not been boiled down but which has fermented also has an extremely positive effect.

Because old urine has a strong odor, you may think it is dirty. Keep in mind that the strong odor is simply ammonia.

Urine which is a few days old undergoes a process of bacterial fermentation; this considerably increases its cleansing and purifying effect. Uric acid is being transmuted into allantoin, a substance with very strong skin-healing capacities.

Urea has a stronger effect if it has been heated. Furthermore, a warm liquid permeates the skin more easily because the pores open up. It is important to realize that our skin is our biggest organ and as it is porous (just like a sieve) it can let things pass through, not only out of the body but into it as well.

1. Massage

Indication: Complementary to fasting; as a treatment of skin disorders; generally as a skin care and rejuvenating tonic; as a substitute for soap.

Urine is massaged into the skin. Massaging can be used for all skin disorders: from a simple rash to eczema and skin cancer. Massaging with urine is a healthy practice even if you do not suffer from a skin disorder, as urine is excellent for skin care. It is also purifying, as it spontaneously produces a natural soap when it comes in contact with skin fat.

This method is vital in the treatment of chronic illnesses and with fasting cures.

An entire body massage with urine takes at least twenty minutes but it is best to massage for at least an hour in case of intensive treatment. For an intensive massage, pour half of the urine into a second dish so that clean urine is available if the first has become dirty. Massage softly and towards the heart, i.e. from the head to the heart and from the feet to the heart. Pay extra attention to the soles of the feet, hands, head, face, back and the areas where the lymph glands are situated, such as the groin and underarms.

Allow at least one hour for the urine to be absorbed. Afterwards, rinse it off with lukewarm water. Do not use soap! Rub a (natural!) lotion into the skin, and the smell of urine will disappear.

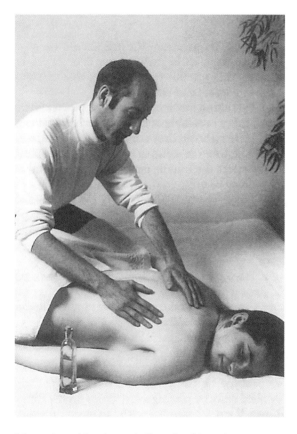

Massaging with urine revitalizes the skin and promotes blood circulation.

Depending on the odor, you may not have to wash the urine off with water. Usually, if it is massaged thoroughly into the skin, its odor is practically gone after a short period of time: the urine has been absorbed into the skin, and the ammonia has evaporated. Whichever method you choose, urine massage takes a bit of getting used to, but is healthy and invigorating.

2. Urine compresses

Indication: Treatment of diseased body parts and internal organs; skin diseases; wounds.

Heat the urine to be used by placing the bottle or pot of urine in a bowl of warm water. Soak a cloth or a piece of cotton wool, depending on the surface to be treated, in the warm urine and place the cloth on the area to be treated. You can also make a compress from a mixture of urine and clay. Old, fresh or boiled urine are suitable for compresses. It is advisable to keep the compresses on the areas to be treated for at least one hour. If desired, refresh the compresses with newly heated urine.

Compresses are recommended for skin disorders where the skin is open or severely swollen. A compress on and around a swelling is better than a urine massage.

This method heals wounds quite effectively, even very large and deep wounds. In Chapter 1, I discussed my positive experience with urine compresses in the treatment of a serious wound on my foot. When I go on vacation, I always keep a bottle of old urine on hand as a first aid remedy for wounds. It works excellently.

Simultaneous compresses on the anus and abdomen are very effective in the treatment of hemorrhoids.

A mixture of clay and urine, applied directly to the skin, can be used in the treatment of skin diseases such as psoriasis.

3. Fresh urine rubbings

Indication: General skin care; bites, rashes and wounds.

For those who value smooth, flawless skin and a healthy appearance, massaging fresh urine daily into the skin in the morning or in the evening is recommended. This is the secret of many a sex symbol and beauty queen. You can use this method during your morning shower. It is also extremely effective as an aftershave lotion. If you can smell the urine after using it as an aftershave, use a (natural) perfumed body or skin lotion.

I rub fresh urine thoroughly into my skin in the morning before I take a shower and pay extra attention to my face and hair. Skin becomes soft and smooth, and hair lustrous and clean.

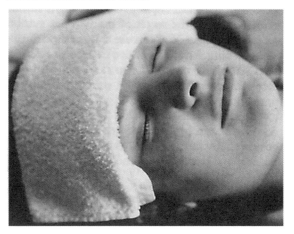

A urine compress.

4. Foot baths and hip baths

Indication: Irritation or fungus infections of the feet; diseases or irritations of genitals or anus; hemorrhoids.

Foot baths are very effective against chilblains and all skin problems on the feet, especially fungus infections or eczema. A foot bath is good for the circulation and can also affect the entire body, as reflex zones are situated under the foot.

Hip baths are recommended for problems of the genitals or on the anus, such as hemorrhoids.

Both heated, old and warm, fresh urine are suitable for these purposes. If you plan to take a foot or hip bath, collect your urine over the course of one day so that you have enough to fill a washtub halfway. You may also dilute the urine with water in order to increase the amount of liquid in the washtub.

5. Scalp and hair massages

Indication: As a general hair care; as a substitute for shampoo; dandruff; hair loss and baldness.

This is an excellent remedy for dandruff, lifeless hair and even baldness and hair loss. Massage urine briskly into the scalp, allow it to be absorbed for thirty minutes to an hour, and then wash it out with lukewarm water (do not use soap or shampoo). Hair becomes clean and lustrous. If you do not rinse out the urine, the effect is even more powerful. However, circumstances do not always allow this. You can use both fresh and old urine for this. The latter shows stronger results.

This method caused my hair to start growing again on a practically bald spot on top of my head. Naturally, this method does not guarantee a new head of hair. Baldness is connected with many factors, which are not always related to the scalp area. Your hair will, however, become more beautiful and vital. Those who apply urine therapy often do not turn grey but retain their original hair colour at a later age. If intensively applied, hair might begin to grow again on bald spots.

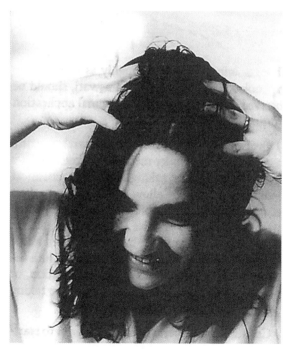

Urine revitalizes and cleanses your hair.

4.5   Warning and Guidelines

WARNING

It is generally not recommended to combine urine therapy with the use of (prescribed) chemical, allopathic medicines or recreational drugs. The combination may be dangerous to your health.

If you are taking any form of allopathic medicine, begin with the external application (urine massage) until you are free of all medication, if possible.

I am often asked what to do when someone is using chemical medicines and also wants to start urine therapy. It is then good first to consider if stopping the medicines would create a life-threatening, dangerous or unbearable situation, or if it would make feel someone very unsafe. If so, start only with external applications and watch very carefully what the reactions are. Then proceed with caution and start internal urine therapy by taking only a few drops urine pure or as a homeopathic tincture. Then gradually build up the amount and keep monitoring the situation.

When the situation improves, you could, after some time, once again, consider if the medicines taken are still necessary.

It is advisable, though, to (gradually) stop using chemical, allopathic drugs that are not strictly necessary. Try to substitute them with natural medicines whenever possible. Natural medicines and urine therapy generally combine very well and often support each other.

IMPORTANT

As with every other natural medicine, urine therapy can bring about a so-called healing crisis. What exactly is a healing crisis? After having ingested urine for some time (depending on your body this can be a day, a week or a month), the body starts to detoxify. In the detoxification period, poisonous substances which have been stored in the body for years are released – substances which may even date back to childhood illnesses. There are a few ways to get rid of these poisonous substances, i.e. through the skin, the intestinal canal, the breath or the mouth and nose. (As already discussed in Chapter 1, the kidneys play a secondary role in the secretion of poisonous substances. Their main purpose is to maintain a healthy balance in the blood.)

The body might also start to fight certain viruses by increasing the temperature and causing a fever.

In short, during the healing crisis, symptoms such as a rash, sweating, fever, pustules, diarrhea, vomiting, headache or coughing may arise. These symptoms usually last no longer than a few hours to a few days. After the crisis you will feel much better and healthier.

Generally, it is recommended not to cease urine therapy during this natural process. If desired, the cure might be (temporarily) continued less intensively. Each person reacts differently, so it is important to listen to your own body. In certain cases it may be wise to stop temporarily and allow the body to take a rest.

The application of urine therapy is not dose-sensitive, i.e. one cannot take an overdose. However, the amount of urine you ingest is obviously connected with the intensity of the healing crisis (the detoxification process), and with the speed of recovery.

A number of practical guidelines for the application of urine therapy follow below. Once again, these are only guidelines. Your own experiences teach you best which method works for you and which does not. Some experience the taste of their urine to be strong and unpleasant or react to it with an intense healing crisis. However, you will probably experience mostly positive results such as an increase in energy and enjoyment, and better health.

The following guidelines, roughly as described in the book *Amaroli* of Dr. S.S. Saraswati, should be observed during every form of internal application of urine therapy:

1) Proceed with caution when starting urine therapy if you are under medical treatment of any kind which involves taking allopathic, chemical medicines. If possible, allow for at least two days between ceasing medication intake and taking urine internally. It is also possible to gradually build up the amount of urine taken by starting with a few drops urine pure or as a homeopathic tincture before you actually stop taking your medication, or in case it is not possible or desirable to stop taking your medication (see above *Warning*).

2) Consult a good therapist or doctor prior to starting urine therapy if you suffer from liver, kidney or heart disease causing serious problems with protein digestion and water balance (for instance if tissue in the legs, arms, abdomen, etc. is swollen from fluids). This also applies if you have high blood pressure. Consult someone who is open to the method of treatment you have chosen.

People with diabetes and kidney diseases can have a very low pH readings. In these cases, always check and correct overacidity before taking urine internally. After necessary adjustments have been made, take only the most alkaline urine as far as drinking is concerned.

3) Proceed more carefully if pus is found in the urine. Only those with a great deal of experience and trust treat infections of the kidneys, bladder or urethra

entirely with urine therapy. Others often choose the method of placing a few drops of urine on the tongue, pure or from an homeopathic tincture, as prescribed in the homeopathic method.

4) While practicing the more intensive form of urine therapy, follow a diet low in protein and salt. Avoid refined, pre-processed and synthetic foods such as sugar, white flour and canned foods. Herbs (also in herbal tea) might cause the urine to taste sharp and bitter, making it more difficult to drink. Some urine therapists advise against drinking milk, primarily because dairy products are processed and contain unnatural additives, and because milk produces a great deal of mucus in the body. In general, it is advisable to decrease the intake of acid-producing foods or food combinations and to increase the intake of alkaline-promoting foods.

(In section *4.6*, I will discuss the influence of food and drink on urine in some more detail.)

5) Reduce the use of alcohol, tobacco and caffeine to an absolute minimum. Urine therapy is most beneficial if your diet contains no alcohol, tobacco products, coffee, junk foods and meat.

6) A healing crisis is a sign that the body is cleansing itself very rapidly and discarding more deep-seated poisonous substances than the excretory system can handle. In this case, the body uses other methods to discard this waste, which may result in unusual reactions. As mentioned above, reduce the amount of urine to be ingested or temporarily stop the treatment and allow the body to rest. Listed below are a number of symptoms which may occur, and how they can be treated.

a) Diarrhea: A day of fasting and complete rest is probably the best measure. Avoid dehydration (especially in countries with a warm climate) by drinking (boiled) water, water with lemon juice or rice water. In this way, the poisonous substances released are better able to find their way out of the body. The second day, eat some rice and yogurt, and by the third day the symptoms should be gone. You can begin the urine therapy again.

b) Skin rash, pustules, etc.: Treat beginning symptoms as follows: rub the infected areas with urine, let the urine soak in for one to two hours and then rinse with water. If this method is not effective, place compresses on the areas. Never squeeze or puncture pustules or blisters. They usually disappear with correct treatment after three to seven days.

c) Vomiting: Vomiting particularly occurs when urine tastes and smells very strong and unpleasant, such as is the case with fever, jaundice and a number of other diseases. In some cases drinking urine can be extremely unpleasant. However, if you drink as much urine as possible, the urine will quickly become thinner and taste more pleasant. Vomiting is good in so far as it cleans the stomach, so there is no cause for worry. After vomiting, you will be less tense and feel better. If vomiting continues even after the stomach is empty, call in professional help. After vomiting out urine, rest and consume only some light liquids, such as water with lemon juice. Once well-rested, continue with urine therapy.

d) Mild fever: A seemingly inexplicable, light fever may occur. Here, the body attempts to burn the poisonous substances released. Fever is actually the most thorough way for the body to discard unwanted substances. Reduce the amount of urine to be ingested, depending on how high the fever is, and get a lot of rest. If necessary, temporarily cease urine therapy until the fever has come down.

e) Coughing and the common cold: During a cleansing process the body sometimes removes excess mucus from the lungs and bronchial tubes. If a great deal of mucus is released, reduce the amount of urine to be ingested or stop temporarily. Start inhaling urine through the nose, as this clears the upper part of the bronchial tubes. Avoid milk and dairy products, as well as all mucus-producing nutrients such as fat and carbohydrates.

f) Overall feeling of weakness: This can occur as a result of the extra energy the body must exert in order to excrete the surplus of poisonous substances.

7) Complete fasting might be too intense, especially if you have been suffering from a chronic illness for a long period of time. In this case, begin urine therapy slowly and step by step. After some time, you might consider a fast consisting of one meal per day. It is always wise to begin slowly rather than diving immediately into deep water only to discover that you cannot swim.

8) During certain illnesses, urine thickens and tastes terribly unpleasant. Drink it anyway, even though this might not be easy. Thick and sharp urine may contain important mineral salts and other valuable substances. Dilute the urine and wash it away with water.

9) Pregnant women can practice urine therapy with the following restrictions. The first morning urine should NOT be ingested. After drinking water, tea or milk, you may drink the second or third flow. The urine should be light in colour, not too sharp or bitter and not too concentrated.

10) Women can drink their urine during their menstruation period. Many women experience this as unpleasant, in which case it is better to stop for a few days. It is always best to consider what feels good for yourself.

11) It is advisable to monitor and balance your pH,

i.e. the acid/alkaline condition of your body, especially with intensive application of urine therapy and fasting. Your urine pH should ideally vary from approximately 5 (more acid) to 8 (more alkaline) during the course of a day. When there is a tendency to either overacidity (acidosis) or overalkalinity (alkalosis), your body is not functioning correctly or your diet is consistently too acid or too alkaline. It is advisable to first try to balance your pH by increasing relaxation, rest, fresh air, exercises and by making dietary adjustments. There are good books available on this subject. You can order pH measuring strips at the pharmacist or drug store.

12) Each person is different, and someone else's experiences do not necessarily apply to you. Age, constitution, physical condition, dietary habits and illness are all contributory factors. Also in your own body the situation constantly changes. Always adjust the application of urine therapy according to what you need and can tolerate at that moment.

13) Trust the process: There are many paths which lead to the same goal of good health.

4.6   *The Influence of Food*

Everything you eat and drink has an effect on your body and consequently on your urine. The healthier your dietary habits are, the better your urine will taste. Urine therapy in itself does not perform miracles. Unless you provide your body with the essential nutrients, it will not possess the raw materials needed to maintain good health.

If you eat healthily and consciously, your urine will contain many essential nutrients which can be re-used. Even so, the body may have a deficiency of certain nutrients if they are not supplemented by a complete range of foods. In the long run, this may result in illnesses and ailments.

How can we prevent this? Where can we get these essential nutrients?

As already discussed, everything we put in or on our body affects the way it functions and performs. The human body is not made to digest and absorb the many harmful additives to which we are nowadays exposed. Chemical products and radiation added to food products have been proven to be harmful.

The recommended range of foods consists of fresh vegetables and fruit, wholemeal grains, seeds, nuts, beans, natural sweeteners such as honey, and a limited use of dairy products.

Alkaline-promoting foods, which deacidify, are particularly recommended. I myself have noted that after an evening meal which consists mainly of raw vegetables, the following morning my urine tastes practically neutral.

It is advisable to follow a vegetarian diet during intensive application of urine therapy. This means that it is best for you to refrain from eating all meat and dairy products, or at least reduce this to a minimum, especially if you practice the therapy for an extended period of time. This also applies if you are fasting or if you drink several glasses of urine per day.

If you continue to eat (large quantities of) meat, you probably have a high concentration of nitrogen wastes, uric acids and other (acidic) substances in your urine, which are not helpful when re-ingested in these large amounts. A surplus of these substances in the blood can lead to an abnormally high degree of acidity. The body consequently 'acidifies', creating a breeding ground for illnesses. The above mentioned substances in high concentrations cause the urine to taste extremely unpleasant. If you wish to keep eating meat, the best meat products are fish and fowl, free of hormones.

Avoid foods containing refined flour products, white sugar and white rice. These nutrients also acidify the blood and body. Avoid processed and radiated foods and foods which contain colorings or flavorings.

A diet can be as personal as you wish. Experiment and consider which diet fits in with your lifestyle and at the same time provides an optimal amount of energy.

Because it is virtually impossible to avoid all poisonous substances, we must take extra precautionary measures concerning our health. Fresh air and clean water are vitally important for good health. Unfortunately, it is not easy to come by good, clean water. Tap water is full of harmful substances, such as fluoride, chlorine and aluminum. It is advisable, especially for drinking, to use purified water from bottles or containers. You can also purchase a good water filter.

It is more difficult to come by fresh air – it is not for sale in bottles or containers... You can, however, go to a wooded area or the beach for the exercise you need. Exercise (in moderation) is important: it increases the heartbeat, stimulates the circulation and strengthens the muscles. It also de-acidifies the blood. Most importantly, it should form a part of your daily routine, and preferably a pleasurable part. Even if you choose to do something different every day, you will benefit from any regular form of exercise.

As already discussed, urine has a healing and nourishing effect on the skin. One can see urine massage as feeding the body through the skin. It also cleans and regenerates. If you want to smell fresh after rubbing urine into your skin, treat your skin with a natural body lotion or oil to which a few drops of essential oil have been added. However, avoid all unnatural body lotions,

creams, etc., since your skin is a very large organ through which substances are absorbed into your body.

As already mentioned, I myself almost never use soap or shampoo, as urine is an excellent cleanser. I also use it as an alternative 'aftershave'. You might also want to experiment with doing without soap and shampoo.

This suggestion gives me the opportunity to make one concluding comment in this section. Although this chapter is full of guidelines and advice, it is important to be aware of what *you* do and why. Take the time to experiment with urine therapy. People learn most of all from their own experiences. Try to feel what a certain method does or means to you. Consider whether it works for you; perhaps it does not work for you at all. Stay in touch with your feelings and your body. It is not only urine therapy which heals you or makes you feel more vital; in the end it is you yourself who is doing that. Urine therapy is an extremely effective aid, especially if you apply it consciously, carefully and with love for yourself.

4.7 Answers to Frequently Asked Questions

1) Isn't urine a waste product which the body excretes because it is poisonous?

The idea that urine is a poisonous waste product is not based upon fact. It has been scientifically proven that, besides water, urine consists mainly of minerals, hormones and enzymes which are not harmful to the body. The body can re-use many of these substances.

Urine is simply a healthy liquid which is filtered out of the bloodstream. What at one moment was part of the blood can be found in urine a split second later.

Certain substances are then filtered by the kidneys and secreted as raw materials which can be directly absorbed by the body upon renewed intake by way of drinking or massaging.

The kidneys filter hundreds of litres of blood per day (approximately 1700 litres). The greatest part of the filtered urine, the so-called 'pre-urine', is directly re-absorbed into the blood. Excess substances and the end products of nitrogen and protein metabolism together with water form the one to two litres of excreted urine.

The kidneys are not intended to remove poisonous substances from the body – the liver, intestines, skin and exhalation take care of this. Obviously, the food you consume finds its way into the blood, and therefore into the urine, which is why it is important to follow a healthy diet. This in itself has nothing to do with urine therapy, but is important if you practice urine therapy.

Even if we assume that poisonous substances can be found in urine, this does not necessarily mean that they are harmful to the body when ingested. If these bodily waste products are natural (i.e., not chemical due to the use of medication, etc.), they can be used to manufacture antibodies which restore balance to the body. In fact, a homeopathic or isopathic effect takes place. Urine is a sort of information card which registers the condition of the blood. When that information is carried back to the body, the body can consequently react according to this feedback and it will normally do this in an appropriate and precise way. In this respect, the body is an extremely advanced and intelligent system. We see how precisely this system works in animals: animals are not in danger of their own poison, as they lick their wounds without any problems. They do not do that just to clean their wounds but also to feed the 'wound information' back into the body so that it can react appropriately.

Furthermore, the intestines do not absorb all the substances we consume and they are able to make a selection. To a certain extent, they select what is useful to the body and excrete the rest through defecation. Certain substances are converted by the bacteria in the intestines into other substances which the body can use or absorb better in that form. Such is the case with urea.

You might ask if urea will not cause any poisoning symptoms when taken in again. Although urea is poisonous when present in very large amounts in the blood, only relatively small amounts of urea are ingested when you drink urine. This does not end up directly in the blood, but rather in the intestines, and primarily has a purifying, cleansing effect. The bulk of it does not show up as urea in the blood, but is converted into the highly useful substance glutamine.

2) Aren't there harmful and pathogenic bacteria in urine?

It is indisputable that the urine from ninety percent of the population is almost entirely free of all bacteria (sterile). Doctors and pathologists confirm this. This is simply because urine does not come into contact with anything until it is excreted, and furthermore contains substances which kill bacteria. In the other ten percent, micro-organisms can be found, which can be caused by a latent illness or infection of the kidneys or urinary passages.

Drinking urine which contains a certain amount of micro-organisms can nevertheless be considered harmless. We constantly eat, drink and inhale bacteria. A large number of bacteria permanently exist in our body, and they generally do not make us sick.

Some caution is suggested with infections of the kidneys, bladder or urinary passages. The number of bacteria can be quite high in these cases and sometimes even pus can be seen in the urine. Even then, some urine therapists, such as Armstrong, recommend drinking everything excreted.

Externally applied, urine is an excellent antiseptic remedy. Fresh urine is sterile and therefore excellent for cleaning wounds. Old urine contains ammonia and other substances which ensure that the infection and decay are combated.

3) If urine is so useful and good for the body, why does the body excrete it?

We can make the comparison here to a dam in a river. If water rises above a certain level, the surplus flows away through the floodgates. However, this does not mean that the surplus water is useless. In the same way, a surplus of water and salts can leave the body at any moment through the kidneys. If you drink more water, more urine is produced and if you drink less water, less urine is produced. Everybody knows this from personal experience.

Nature works in cycles, allowing matter to return to its original substance and be re-used for construction. Many substances still floating through the blood in compounded form are filtered by the kidneys and return to their original substances. In this way they can easily be re-absorbed by the body.

Once again, I refer to the example of a tree which lives off its fallen leaves. Nature possesses an infallible capacity for recycling, of which urine therapy is a remarkable, but sadly forgotten, example.

I would again like to point out that we have all experienced this urine cycle as a foetus in the womb. For almost nine months, we drank our own urine in the form of amniotic fluid. This liquid was an important contribution to the development of our bodies. Drinking urine is certainly not strange. On the contrary, it is the foundation of our existence.

4) If drinking our own urine is so natural and useful, why hasn't nature equipped us with an instinct to do this automatically?

Rational thinking has completely suppressed many natural human instincts. For example, all animals avoid eating if they are sick. Many illnesses can be quickly cured in this way, since digesting food requires a great deal of energy. By not eating, we can direct much more energy towards the recovery process.

Human beings, however, often continue eating when they are sick. On top of that, the patient is often advised to eat especially well, even if he or she is absolutely not hungry.

Sick or wounded animals instinctively use their own bodily fluids. By licking their wounds, for example, they not only keep the wound clean, but also send a signal to the body, which reacts to this 'self-injection'. Goats sometimes urinate directly into their own mouths, and many other animals (e.g. dogs) lick the urine from others of their species.

We have obviously strayed quite far from our instincts in other areas as well. It is certainly not instinctual to light a cigarette or consume alcohol.

It is therefore safer to assume that nature has equipped us with a number of instincts, but that we, as people, have largely lost contact with them.

5) Isn't it true that urine therapy seems to be effective, but that the simultaneous change of dietary habits is actually the healing factor?

Of course dietary habits greatly influence your health. Urine therapy and healthy dietary habits go together. As already mentioned, no substance which has not earlier been consumed will appear in the urine. A change in dietary habits as part of urine therapy undoubtedly plays an important role in a possible healing process.

Actually, urine therapy is also effective for those who already have healthy dietary habits and yet for one reason or another get sick. Furthermore, the rate at which symptoms improve when you apply urine therapy is remarkably higher than when you exclusively change your dietary habits. Urine therapy also has an extraordinarily positive effect if you fast exclusively on water and urine, in which case you completely refrain from eating. Furthermore, the same results are achieved with a urine and water fast in one week as with a juice or water fast in two to three weeks.

The fact remains: the substances you eat, drink or otherwise ingest are indeed important, especially regarding long-term health. Applying urine therapy while maintaining unhealthy dietary habits is like lighting a candle to the sun.

As a closing remark, there are no unequivocal rules regarding a healthy diet and lifestyle. This is very personal and usually, deep down, you know best what is best for you.

6) Can't the effects of urine therapy be attributed to suggestion or belief?

Those who seek refuge in urine therapy as a 'last resort' have often already made the rounds by every other method of treatment, from allopathy to homeopathy, Ayurveda, etc. They hoped and believed these other therapies would work. Yet it seems that many who did not achieve results with other methods of treatment have been cured by urine therapy. This is remarkable when you consider that the nature and obscurity of urine therapy initially evoke a skeptical reaction.

In India, I spoke with a urine therapist who, in his role as supervisor at a national park, also successfully treated animals with urine therapy. Here, there is no question of the treated animal under the influence of suggestion or belief.

However, it is generally important to believe in the method of treatment you choose. This is also true if you choose another treatment.

7) Doesn't urine taste disgusting?

Our aversion to urine is the result of preconceptions and conditioning. We have been taught that urine is dirty. In reality, urine usually does not taste dirty. Many who have been drinking it for some time even think it tastes and smells pleasant.

The taste of urine partly depends on what you have eaten and drunk the previous day. If you eat a great deal of animal proteins, use a lot of spices or drink strong herbal tea, your urine will probably have a strong taste. Also, when your body is out of balance, i.e. if you are sick, urine often tastes stronger than normal. While applying urine therapy it is wise to reduce the intake of especially animal proteins and strong herbs and spices.

If you wish to gradually become accustomed to the taste, mix urine with water or fruit juice or mix a spoonful of honey into the urine.

In general, taste is subjective. What is delicious to one person is disgusting to another. Furthermore, your taste can change with time. Most people who drink beer or wine for the first time in their life think it tastes disgusting, but after some time they get used to the taste and actually enjoy it. The same is true for olives, blue cheese, etc.

Regarding medicine, it is interesting to note that people are willing to ingest the most disgusting tasting drinks and pills as long as a doctor prescribes it.

Likewise, if you are sick, you might also try to overcome your resistance to the taste of urine. But do it with love.

8) If urine therapy was so popular in the past, as is maintained, why are people no longer interested in it, and why don't they know it can be useful?

With the development of culture and technological progress, we have strayed further and further from nature. Our interest in natural medicines, including urine therapy, has therefore decreased. Furthermore, in many respects we have turned away from our own bodies. This has made urine therapy psychologically inaccessible to us; in other words, we think our own bodily products are disgusting.

Our economic system is based upon scarcity, and scarcity is related to dependence. Urine therapy provides 'patients' with so much independence that the remedy, urine, is not lucrative. Urine is free and always available for those who need it. In a world in which money talks, urine therapy can appear to be threatening to those who earn their living by manufacturing or prescribing medicine. In short, urine therapy does not fit in the current economic picture of scarcity.

Many people believe we are healthier nowadays thanks to advances in medical science. This is partly true. The flip side of the coin is that we have had to give up a great deal of freedom and independence. The enormous efforts of medical science are partly based upon the failure to really cure illnesses. Fighting symptoms is considered to be crucial, but this does not take care of the cause. Urine therapy, being a real nature cure, not only reduces the symptoms, but also deals with the cause of the illness.

Keep in mind that urine therapy is not a 'wonder drug' that relieves all symptoms. Illness always has several causes and is usually not only physical. Feelings, thoughts and the environment also play a role. If you apply urine therapy in order to get rid of a symptom, but after improvement continue to treat yourself and your body carelessly, the symptoms might reappear. It is therefore important to also pay attention to other factors playing a role in the healing process.

9) How do acquaintances and friends react when you tell them that you drink your urine? Is it not better to keep quiet about it?

Nowadays, the taboos surrounding bodily excretions are great. We consider many things to be dirty as soon as they leave our body, and forget that those same substances just a few minutes before were an integral part of our body. Everybody knows that the best way to get a laugh is by telling jokes about peeing and shitting. I get the whole range of reactions whenever I talk about my experiences. This is how we have been brought up, and although I take urine therapy seriously, I generally prefer an approach with a healthy dose of humour.

However, if you feel uncomfortable about telling it to those around you, but still want to experiment with urine therapy, feel free to do this without mentioning it to others. When you are convinced it works for you, the reluctance to talk about it will gradually subside, and maybe even disappear. Perhaps you will start to enjoy talking about it, as I do. You can be sure that you will be surrounded by plenty of laughter, which in fact can be rather pleasant. An old saying maintains that it is good to combine what is useful with what is pleasurable; you can be sure of that with urine therapy!

It is a different matter if you have difficulties explaining urine therapy to your immediate family or partner. Support from those closest to you is essential. Thorough explanation can work wonders. Let them read this book. Before you know it, their interest in urine therapy will outweigh their aversion.

As for the smell, it is not as strong as one would expect. With a little bit of care, those closest to you will not notice a thing. The odor of urine is much less repulsive than most people think since most associate urine with public toilets. Actually, it often smells rather pleasant when applied fresh on the skin. I myself regularly use pure urine as aftershave and hair lotion, and nobody has ever told me I smell dirty. If I suspect that I smell of urine, I use a natural, fresh-smelling cream or skin lotion and the problem disappears.

There will always be people who think it is bizarre or dirty. It is up to you to decide what is more important to you: your own good health or other people's opinions.

10) For which illnesses is urine therapy effective and for which is it ineffective? Are there any contra-indications?

In theory, urine therapy is effective for every illness. Actually, a diagnosis is unnecessary prior to applying urine therapy. This therapy is a total treatment aimed at strengthening or recovering the balance in the body. Because there are countless ways in which the balance can be upset, there are also countless illnesses. Medical science has conveniently categorized and named these illnesses. Urine therapy is a very personal treatment and can be applied in many ways. Likewise, an imbalance in the body can occur in countless ways and on different levels. Because the application of urine therapy does not require medication which goes with a certain symptom, a diagnosis is also unnecessary.

Nevertheless, because we are so accustomed to receiving a diagnosis, it is for most of us reassuring to know which 'label' is attached to our illness. Furthermore, this can also help us in choosing other natural remedies, and these can certainly be used

simultaneously with urine therapy. The treatments often support each other. In the *Damar Tantra*, of which the entire document can be found in Chapter 7 of this book, combinations of herbal mixtures and urine are often prescribed.

Urine therapy can be applied at all times and for every illness, although in a number of cases extra attention and caution are advised. This applies especially if pus is found in the urine, indicating that the urine contains many bacteria. It might then be wiser to ingest only a few drops of urine, which will have a homeopathic or isopathic effect. In the case of chronic illness, constantly keep an eye on your general condition, especially if your body is already weak. An illness such as diabetes requires extra precaution, in particular with respect to the accompanying diet.

Furthermore, pay attention to the degree of acidity of the blood and urine. If the blood is too acidic, the urine might also be rather acidic, which may cause irritations during application. Reduce the degree of acidity by fasting, taking natural medicines and following an appropriate diet (low in protein and vegetarian).

So, there are no contra-indications, but there are certainly conditions under which urine therapy can best be applied. Once again, one very important condition is the quality and combination of your diet.

11) Why is it particularly recommended to drink the morning urine?

The majority of useful, vital substances is found in the morning urine. This is because at night, while you sleep, your body is totally relaxed. This deep relaxation gives the body the chance to carry out its recovery activities'. The decomposition products partly end up in the urine and can be re-absorbed and used for new build-up processes. This process of filtering by the kidneys returns the so-called raw decomposition products to their original substances, which can subsequently be re-absorbed and re-used by the body.

Certain hormones are also released during sleep, a number of which are intended to bring about the above mentioned deep relaxation. Re-absorbing these hormones ensures that we are more rested during the waking hours. Moreover, it saves the body energy because it does not have to manufacture these hormones again.

Furthermore, ingestion of the morning urine, which is full of hormones, regulates the entire hormonal process. Some of these hormones have the particular function of maintaining hormonal balance. I know a woman who accurately kept track of her menstruation cycle for quite some time while she was planning her pregnancy. Once she started practicing urine therapy, her cycle was suddenly completely constant, compared with the fluctuations and deviations she had previously observed.

12) Should you only use your own urine?

In theory, it is best to use exclusively your own urine, especially if internally applied. However, if you are in a state of shock and cannot urinate, the urine from somebody else can safely be administered. If possible, use the urine from somebody of the same sex. Different hormones can be found in the urine from a male than in that of a female.

For certain illnesses, it seems to be beneficial to ingest the urine from children. The urine from a child is often very pure, especially if the child follows a healthy diet. In some cases, the urine from a child can also be used in the external massage application for the seriously ill who cannot produce enough of their own urine.

It is certainly possible to use the urine from another person for massage.

The urine from pregnant women is also recommended by some urine therapists in the treatment of certain symptoms, but further research is necessary before we can say more about this.

According to the latest reports, it is almost certain that HIV cannot be transmitted through urine.

Urine from different people usually does not differ much in its ingredients, which is why the urine from one person will also to some extent work for somebody else. However, your own urine contains personal, characteristic substances and provides the particular information the body needs in order to carry out the healing process as effectively as possible.

13) What about using nutritional supplements such as vitamins etc., when practicing urine therapy?

In general, it is no problem to combine urine therapy with any other form of natural treatment. This also applies to the use of nutritional supplements as long as they are natural. On should refrain from any chemically manufactured supplements.

Experience has shown that the use of vitamin supplements in combination with the practice of urine therapy can considerably cut down the amount of supplements you need to take, because of the recycling effect. Many substances, such as vitamins and enzymes, act as carriers for other substances, and after having fulfilled their task they leave the body unaltered. Thus they can be used and taken in again to carry out the same job.

Some vitamin supplements contain very high doses of specific vitamins. This can make the urine look very dark and taste and smell very strong. However, this is not a problem, although it might be somewhat unpleasant to drink.

14) What do you do, if you can't get over the taste?

When it is not possible for you to get used to the taste, there are several other ways in which you can take urine into your body. Massaging with urine allows urine to be absorbed into the body through the skin. As far as taking urine in through the mouth, one could dilute it with a lot of water, apple juice, etc.; one could take just a few drops mixed in juice, tea or other fluids; one could make use of a homeopathic tincture or an injection.

To help make the taste of your urine more acceptable, it is wise to experiment with your diet. It is recommended to eat lots of fruits and fresh vegetables and cut down on meat, spices, dairy products and carbohydrates. Fruits and vegetables form a healthy diet anyway, and they normally make the urine taste milder and more watery. It is then usually easier to drink your urine.

For people who feel either occasionally or permanently a strong disgust blocking them from drinking their own urine, I would suggest that it may be worth first trying to discover their personal, psychological relation to urine. Clearing up some deeper issues surrounding body secretions might help to overcome the aversion.

5. A NATURAL PHARMACY: Medical and Scientific Aspects of Urine Therapy

5.1 In Search of an Explanation

Over the years, urine therapy has proved to be an effective tool for healing. Most urine therapists, some of whom have been practicing urine therapy for decades, have never sought an explanation for why it works: their own experiences were sufficient proof. For some time now, however, there has been increasing interest in the search for a scientific explanation. This is because urine therapists believe it is important for urine therapy to be acknowledged as a valid method of treatment: doctors should be well-informed about the effects of this therapy so that as many people as possible can benefit from it. Since members of the medical world demand an explanation, the interest in scientific research has grown.

Another reason for this growing interest is that a number of 'mainstream' doctors have also had positive experiences with urine therapy, which is reason enough for them to investigate how and why it works.

This is not a recent development: in the 1930s, for example, the German pediatrician Martin Krebs successfully treated many patients with urine therapy, and subsequently published the results (see bibliography). As a physician, he was convinced that urine therapy was an effective method of treatment, but he also realized that other doctors would not readily accept this fact since it conflicted with the scientific dogma which formed the foundation of their profession.

In order to be able to acknowledge urine therapy as an effective method of treatment, a number of doctors within the medical world are now interested in how it works. Discovering how it actually works, however, will not be easy. Random, double-blind, cross-over research could be useful, but is difficult to execute. It requires that several groups of 'test patients' are involved in the research, and that neither the patients nor those executing the treatment know whether 'the remedy' (urine) is being used – only those leading the research know this. This type of research is perfectly easy to conduct with pills (since all pills look alike), but is somewhat more difficult with urine. Although double-blind, cross-over research is considered to be the most valuable way to discover if a certain method of treatment is effective, there are also other reliable research methods. One of these is to observe and document urine therapy treatments, and to conduct more research into the benefits of urine as a therapeutic substance, both in terms of its separate components and as a total entity.

Some people doubt the effectiveness of urine therapy and therefore do not yet acknowledge the value of this research. A relevant point here is that the highest placebo-effect, i.e. the positive effect of a treatment solely because the patient believes it works (even if it does not), is 30%.[1] If the treatment produces a much higher percentage of improvement, the therapy should be given the benefit of the doubt.

This certainly seems to be the case with urine therapy. The literature reveals that the majority of people who use urine therapy consistently and 'according to the rules' believe they have benefited from it. It is true that the literature on urine therapy is often written by enthusiastic urine therapists. It is therefore important to be critical of the often expressed opinion that urine therapy, if correctly applied, has never caused negative side effects. This applies likewise to the assertion that very few people have experienced no noteworthy improvement from practicing urine therapy. Taking this into account, however, the percentage of positive results still seems to be far above 30%, sufficient reason to give urine therapy the deserved benefit of the doubt and to conduct further research.

As stated above, a good deal of research has already been conducted within the medical world into the composition of urine and its separate components. The researchers Free and Free published a report listing two hundred substances found in urine. They point out that these are only the most significant substances, and that urine probably contains thousands of components.[2] Several substances found in urine seem to be of value as medication, some of which have already been processed and used.

A number of substances found in urine are briefly discussed in this chapter. References to the relevant research articles can be found in the notes at the end of this chapter. Since this book is not intended to be a scientific publication, many references have simply been reproduced in good faith from other publications. The references should be seen mainly as a starting point for those who wish to conduct further research into this material.

The fact that certain individual components of urine are effective does not prove that urine therapy is effective. Conversely, however, it can be assumed that the components which have a particular effect as an individual substance, have the same effect when taken as a component of urine. In certain cases it could be imagined that the combination of these substances with other components of urine reduces or cancels out the effectiveness, but this is not the most obvious conclusion. We can, therefore, reasonably assume that if an individual substance displays a certain characteristic, it will also have this characteristic as a component of urine. The more individually effective substances found in urine, the stronger the argument that urine as a total entity has a therapeutic effect.

A condition of this argument is that urine as a total entity does not contain substances with an obviously harmful effect: as yet there is no evidence to suggest that such substances have been found in urine. The small amounts of poisonous substances which can be found in urine largely seem to have a positive effect on the immune system (see below). If urine did contain extremely harmful substances, it would be impossible to explain how many people (myself included) who drink their own urine every day for years could still be in exceptionally good health.

So research has not yet been conducted on urine as a total entity which can be therapeutically applied. Still unanswered are questions regarding how and why urine therapy works, since urine is used here as a total entity. A number of hypotheses have, however, been suggested which can serve as the basis for further scientific research.

According to Dr. Bartnett, applying urine therapy using self-produced urine can be considered to be an extension of the methods of Jenner and Pasteur.[3] An important task of the immune system is to rid the human body of diseased or unusable substances that have developed during the course of an illness. When these substances reach healthy tissue, the serum or blood becomes stronger, the activity of leucocytes (white blood cells) increases, and the patient probably recovers. This phenomenon is known as auto-inoculation or self-vaccination and can be seen as mother nature's method of healing an illness without external intervention.

Urine therapy can also be seen as a form of self-vaccination: certain bodily substances which have been removed from the body, some of which may have been produced as a result of illness, are re-introduced into the body in small amounts. These substances are re-absorbed into the blood through either the intestines or the skin. According to this hypothesis, the immune system is then given the chance to react appropriately.

The doctors Remington, Merler and Uhr have demonstrated that a particular part of urine-protein is able to eliminate certain pathogens.[4] This discovery supports the assumption that urine therapy can be used to treat or prevent certain illnesses.

In the early nineteenth century, Dr. Charles Duncan conducted research into therapies with self-produced substances, including urine therapy.[5] He demonstrated that patients suffering from gonorrheic urethritis (infection of the urinary tube as a result of the venereal disease gonorrhea) produce their own medication in the form of their own discharge. Auto-therapy was applied here by placing a drop of a patient's discharge

directly on the tongue, in order to stimulate the body's natural powers. This method had a strong healing effect at every stage of the illness: if applied at an early stage, it could cause the gonorrhea to disappear.

Auto-therapy is based on the principle that the body can use all fresh, self-produced, unaltered diseased tissue substances which originate from the microorganisms causing the illness. Seen in this light, patients have their own medication in exactly the form constructed by nature to heal their condition.

The results of Dr. William D. Linscott's research suggest that auto-therapy strengthens and stimulates the immune system, in particular with regard to the T-cells. The T-cell population of several patients who initially displayed a low T-cell count increased after treatment with urine therapy.[6]

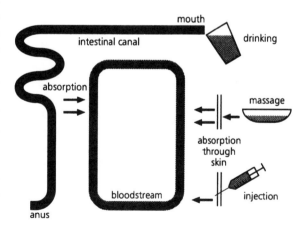

Urine therapy: a form of self-vaccination. Vital substances are re-absorbed by means of drinking, massage, injection, etc.

5.2 Several Hypotheses

A number of possible explanations (hypotheses) as to how and why urine therapy works are presented in the literature. In the book *Amaroli* of Dr. S.S. Saraswati (see bibliography), eight hypotheses are clearly listed. These should not be seen as eight separate hypotheses: the authors believe that several factors combine to give urine therapy its exceptional effectiveness. They also believe that each of these factors should first be examined, researched and tested separately.

Amaroli does not discuss the potentially important role of urea. More information about urea has recently become available, largely from research conducted by the natural doctor and chiropractor John Wynhausen and by Martha M. Christy.[7] This information is significant since doctors often argue that urea is highly poisonous. I have therefore added an additional hypothesis which focuses on the role of urea in urine therapy.

I have added another hypothesis concerning a scientifically controversial subject. Considering the alchemical and spiritual context in which urine therapy often appears, it might very well be that the effect of urine therapy can partly be attributed to the process of transmutation. The theory of transmutation is based on the idea that certain substances can be transformed within the body into other substances. This theory belongs to the area of a new, holistic paradigm and does not fit in with the old, strictly mechanistic paradigm as far as the body and its functions are concerned.

The ten resulting hypotheses concerning the effective factors in urine therapy treatment are presented briefly below. Once again, these are merely hypotheses and should be seen as a starting point for further research.

They are presented as mere hypotheses here because no research has yet been conducted to test them and therefore nothing has been scientifically proven.

The ten hypotheses relate to the following ten areas:

1. *Re-absorption and re-use of nutrients*
2. *Re-absorption of hormones*
3. *Re-absorption of enzymes*
4. *Re-absorption of urea*
5. *Immunological effect*
6. *Bactericidal and virucidal effect*
7. *Salt therapy*
8. *Diuretic effect*
9. *Transmutation theory*
10. *Psychological effect*

1. Re-absorption and re-use of nutrients

The assertion that urine can cure illnesses *because* it contains minerals, vitamins and other nutrients which are essential for one's health is not entirely accurate. We obtain these substances in sufficient quantities from the food we eat, assuming that we follow a healthy, well-balanced diet. By drinking or massaging with urine, we possibly re-use and re-absorb a number of vitamins, amino acids, salts, hormones, etc. as nutrients.

This can be especially important during illness, when diseased body tissue enters the blood and must therefore be excreted. The filtering process in the kidneys should break down this tissue to its original materials, after which it can be re-used by the body to build up new tissue.

The composition of urine changes during illness, because certain essential substances do not reach their intended destination and are subsequently filtered out by the kidneys. A good example of this is liver blockage, which can result in hepatitis (inflammation of the liver). If a blockage develops in the liver, bile produced by the liver cannot reach the intestinal canal, instead seeps into the blood and subsequently ends up in the urine, resulting in weakness and nausea. The shortage of bile in the digestive tract restricts the digestion of fats and proteins. Rest and a diet low in fats and proteins are usually prescribed.[8]

However, the substance which should digest these proteins and fats can be found in the urine in precisely the correct amount. According to this theory, the application of urine therapy allows bile and other liver enzymes to be re-used instead of wasted.

This is just one example of an illness in which important substances can be re-used via the urine. Research could also be conducted for other illnesses concerning the way in which important bodily substances can be saved and re-used.

2. *Re-absorption of hormones*

As stated above, many hormones end up in the urine. The basis for this hypothesis is that we can re-introduce these into the body by drinking or massaging with urine.

Since proteins are harmed by the acids, pepsins and enzymes in the digestive tract, the hormones re-absorbed into the body if one drinks urine will mainly be the small ones which are not proteins (protein-complexes). The sex hormones, adrenal gland hormones and thyroid hormones will almost certainly be re-absorbed, the effects of which need to be more closely researched. The external application of urine to the skin allows hormones to be re-absorbed by the body without being destroyed. Massaging with urine is therefore an important complementary component of urine therapy, as urine

is directly absorbed into the tissue.[9] Enemas are also a good way to prevent destruction of certain hormones by gastric juices, which is why this method often helps cure allergic disorders better than when urine is orally ingested. The same applies for urine injections.

Re-absorption can be of value in two ways. Firstly, certain hormones have a very specific effect during a healing process. For example, corticosteroids secreted by the adrenal cortex inhibit infections and have a positive effect in the treatment of allergies such as asthma and hay fever, skin disorders such as eczema and psoriasis, and inflammatory illnesses such as rheumatism. Urine therapy has proved to be an extremely effective aid in the treatment of all these illnesses, but it has not yet been demonstrated that these hormones play a part in the treatment. The word 'proved' as used here indicates observation of a particular treatment and the results, and the logical conclusions that can be drawn.

Secondly, re-absorption can be a means for the body to generally conserve energy: re-ingestion of hormones gives the body the chance to re-use at least a number of these, so that it is not necessary to expend energy on manufacturing new hormones.

Hormones are actually extremely powerful molecules, the production of which requires a great deal of energy. Once produced, they are able to cause a complete alteration in the balance of bodily processes, the personality, the emotions and the state of mind, even if only a few molecules are released. So even the slightest re-absorption of hormones may well have a powerful effect on our state of health and level of energy.[10]

I have already referred to research on the effects of melatonin, a hormone found in urine which possibly has a calming effect.[11] Melatonin also has a powerful anti-cancer effect.[12]

It is quite possible that the sages of olden times were well aware of the hormonal effects of urine. They state that if a person is unable to urinate, the urine from somebody of the same sex is acceptable, but not from somebody of the other sex.

Although cultural and social factors could have played a part in this rule, the fact is that female urine contains considerably greater amounts of female hormones, such as oestrogen. If ingested over a long period of time by a man, this could have a feminizing effect. The opposite is true for a woman who ingests male urine.

Some people recommend to use the first urine after sexual intercourse. During the process of sexual stimulation certain hormones are released in the higher endocrinal glands which have a regenerating effect on the body. This applies for men as well as women.[13]

3. Re-absorption of enzymes

Urine contains many enzymes, which might explain why urine therapy is effective against arteriosclerosis, heart attack, pulmonary embolism, etc. Based on research conducted on the enzyme Urokinase, positive results can be expected from the effects of enzymes in urine as a 'total entity'. Urokinase causes vasodilation and resembles nitroglycerine in its ability to strengthen the bloodstream from the coronary artery to the cardiac muscle. Urokinase is extracted from urine and brought on the market as medicine on a large scale.[14]

Other enzymes are probably active in urine, but more specific information is not yet available.

4. Re-absorption of urea

The following information is partly derived from a research report as recently presented by John Wynhausen at the First All India Conference on Urine Therapy.[15]

Besides water, urea is the main component of urine and is a decomposition product of converted proteins. A person excretes approximately an average of 25 to 30 grams of urea per day. We come in contact with urea at an early age, i.e. as a foetus in the womb. The level of urea in amniotic fluid, which consists for the most part of urine from the foetus, doubles in the last two months of pregnancy.[16] Before we are born, we drink well over half a litre per day of this liquid. The foetus also 'breathes' it in – this is essential for proper development of the lungs. Scars disappear after an operation on a foetus in the womb due to the healing capacities of the urea in the amniotic fluid.[17]

It is still unclear whether urea in amniotic fluid is converted into another substance when taken in by the foetus. This is probably not the case, since bacteria are not yet active in the intestinal canal.

Once we are born, the intestinal flora start to work, which have a special role in the conversion of urea. Scientists estimate that 25% of the urea in an adult finds its way into the intestines, where it is decomposed into ammonia by intestinal bacteria.[18] Some of this ammonia ends up in the liver, where part of it is converted into urea, and another part is converted into glutamine, an extremely useful amino acid.[19] The liver converts a great deal of the ammonia, in theory poisonous, into other substances. Although ammonia is highly poisonous even in moderate amounts, this small amount is extremely important: it regulates the pH-value of the blood and has a powerful anti-viral effect.[20]

If it were true that the urea concentration increases the more often a person drinks urine, we would expect urine to become stronger or more bitter-tasting. However, the opposite is true: urine becomes more watery and less bitter, which suggests that urea is converted. It is quite possible that urea is indeed converted into glutamine by ammonia. As described above, this process takes place in the intestinal canal.

Research demonstrates the vital importance of glutamine in the maintenance and construction of specialized tissue, such as in the brain, the small intestine and in the growth and activity of the mucous membrane of the intestinal canal. Glutamine has a healing effect on ulcers and wounds in the intestinal canal.[21] The most important function of glutamine, however, is its ability to strengthen the immune system,[22] and could be an important key in explaining why urine therapy is such a successful method of treatment. The body re-uses a certain part of urea; the extra supply created by applying urine therapy increases the glutamine level in the body. This consequently strengthens the immune system and specialized organs, and at the same time heals damages to the digestive tract.

Urea, in so far as it is not decomposed, also affects the brain and central nervous system. High doses of urea are sometimes administered during brain surgery in order to temporarily shrink the brain, which is necessary for opening the skull.[23] Less than one tenth of such a dose is ingested when a person drinks urine. Nevertheless, this small amount also brings about a slight reduction of pressure in the brain and spinal cord. John Wynhausen, a chiropractor, is well aware of the health problems caused by too much pressure on the skull and vertebrae. Wynhausen sees this, at least on a physical level, as one of the most important causes of human illness at this time. Seen in this light, drinking urine, and consequently a regular decrease in pressure, yields extremely positive results.

Urea is also successfully administered in rather high doses to patients with sickle cell anemia, an extremely painful and supposedly incurable illness.[24] Research and experience have demonstrated that, if administered daily in four doses of approximately 40 grams, urea has a healing and preventive effect. This also indicates that the body can endure high doses of urea without displaying negative side effects.

A third noteworthy application of urea can be found in the treatment of cancer by Professor Dr. Danopoulos.[25] He experimented with injecting urea mixed with a saline solution in and around skin cancer and as a treatment for breast cancer. He also conducted research on drinking urea dissolved in water in order to fight liver cancer, and reported positive results. Danopoulos then began combining urea with creatine hydrate, another component of urine, and in this way successfully treated other kinds of cancer. Urea also seems to be quite effective in fighting bladder cancer. You might wonder how bladder cancer can arise if urea, constantly present in the bladder, is such an effective anti-cancer remedy. However, bladder cancer is a relatively rare form of cancer and generally only found in those who work with certain poisonous chemicals. Perhaps the effect of urea is counteracted or cancelled out by these chemicals. Further research on this topic is necessary.

Urea also plays an extremely important role in the external application of urine, as it helps transport hormones through the skin. Many hormones are destroyed by the enzymatic system of the digestive system if urine is internally applied. Hormones can probably return to the body in their original form if urine is administered 'through the skin'. Moreover, a 'transdermal' administration ensures that hormones are absorbed into the body slowly and in specific portions, which significantly increases the effectiveness of such a minimal amount of urine.

Urea has the capacity to moisten the skin and regulate its condition, one of the reasons why it is processed in many skin creams. Some pharmaceutical companies use horse urine for the production of urea and they actually have lots of horses in their factory, just for this purpose, I have been told recently.[26]

Other research data concerning urea are:

Urea is an oxidizing substance which ensures that the disintegrating proteins (proteins in the area of a wound or inflammation) dissolve. If urea is present, disintegrating tissue cannot feed itself with other rotting material. It dissolves fats and other natural bodily secretions. Urea is even more effective when heated.[27]

Due to its strong anti-bacterial nature, urine has an inhibitive effect on the growth of tuberculosis bacilli. Bacteria-inhibiting or bacteria-killing effects of urine increase with a decreasing pH. Urea and ammonia, closely related, play an important role here.[28] When brought in contact with urea, complex polymers are transformed or decomposed into monomers, which can then be endured by the body.[29]

For further information on the bactericidal effects of urea, see also section 6. *Bactericidal and virucidal effect* and its notes. Urea has also been used in the treatment of kidney failure and uremic conditions with positive results.[30]

5.   *Immunological effect*

Clearly urine is not toxic, although some toxic substances might be present in urine in small amounts, especially if one is ill. This small amount of toxic substances possibly contributes to the effectiveness of urine therapy. If toxic substances enter the body, the body's defense mechanisms are called into action (the defense or immune system). If substances which leave the body via the urine are the same as those involved in the illness process, they can stimulate the defense system to attack and in this way fight the illness. This might explain why urine therapy has proven so helpful in treating allergies.[31]

A similar process takes place when a person is vaccinated against certain diseases, in which case a small amount of poisonous substances is injected into a healthy body. This stimulates the immune system to manufacture antibodies (and thus defend the body), and could be called a homeopathic or isopathic effect. We have already extensively dealt with this subject in the section covering Armstrong's ideas. The practice of drinking and massaging with urine allows antibodies greater access to the body, which stimulates the immune system. I refer to Linscott's research, as mentioned in section *5.1*, on auto-therapy and an increase of T-cells (see note *6*).

The possible significance of urea and glutamine for the immune system is discussed in section *4. Re-absorption of urea*.

Abele suggests that the presence of antigens and antibodies in urine strengthens the immune system when urine is re-introduced into the body. The re-introduction of small amounts of bacteria or parasites found in urine may stimulate the production of IgE. IgA (a virus inhibiting substance that prevents micro-organisms from becoming embedded in the mucous) also plays a role here. IgA is found in mucous and in excretion products, and therefore also in urine. Urine therapy increases the production of IgA, which possibly explains why this therapy has a positive effect on infections of the urinary passages and the kidneys while other treatments offer little relief.[32]

Several studies demonstrate that antibodies against for example salmonella, diphtheria, poliomyelitis and HIV can be found in urine.[33]

6. Bactericidal and virucidal effect

Although it is not yet entirely clear why urine has a germicidal and antiseptic effect, it is known that urea plays an important role here. Ammonia and salt also have a similar purifying effect. Besides killing bacteria, urine also inhibits or destroys various viruses and fungi. Scientific research has demonstrated that both urea and ammonia have a powerful anti-viral effect.[34]

Applying urine to a fresh cut or scrape prevents infection and keeps flies away (important in countries with a warm climate). Urine compresses from fresh or old urine help to combat infections and often cause them to disappear. Although urine does not entirely prevent the growth of bacteria in the urethra (infections often arise), it clearly has a powerful antiseptic effect when externally applied.

Herz also successfully treated infections of the urinary passages with urine therapy. The positive results can be traced back to the stimulating effect of the re-ingested urine on the immune system. As discussed above, in such a case, IgA is produced in greater quantities.[35]

7. Salt therapy

Drinking salt water serves as an important therapeutic remedy during certain (fasting) cures. Salt water is also frequently applied in yoga to clean the body thoroughly from within and it relieves such illnesses as asthma, stomach ulcer, indigestion and constipation. Drinking urine, which is also a salt substance, has the same effect. This could be an important reason for its success as a therapeutic remedy.

Salt solutions remove old mucous embedded in the mucous membranes. If one drinks a salt liquid, part of the salt goes into the body, where it dissolves the surplus of mucous in the lungs and in other organs.

According to those who work with this therapy, warm salt water, and in this sense also fresh, warm urine, is particularly useful during illnesses in which the body does not generate enough heat to keep the normal bodily secretions thin and watery. Moreover, urine draws out surplus fluid from mucous which has become too watery due to an illness. This also explains why compresses of warm, concentrated urine externally applied are so effective.

As a salt liquid, urine also has a laxative effect and is recommended to relieve constipation. As it moves through the intestinal canal, the salt detaches waste and draws water into the intestines, as a result of which bowel movement becomes easier.

According to this theory, drinking urine, like drinking salt water, accelerates the metabolism. It removes a surplus of sugar from the blood and draws out toxic substances from cells. In this way, urine therapy is a good cleansing technique.

According to urine therapists, urine has an extra advantage above salt water because urine contains a small amount of natural cortisone. This brings us back to the possible hormonal effects of urine.

Using urine instead of salt is also more effective because urea and ammonia are organic solvents: they dissolve fats and other natural bodily secretions. These substances probably ensure that the mucous membranes and body cells are powerfully affected.

Dabbing with salt water usually helps clean wounds; urine has the same effect. Urine is more effective than salt water because it contains healing substances such as allantoin (see section *5.3 Some Individual Substances Found in Urine*).

8. Diuretic effect

According to this theory, urine therapy ensures that

the kidneys work more quickly and that the body is stimulated to produce more urine. Metabolic products composed of proteins such as urea, nitrogen and ammonia are excreted out of the body via the urine as soon as there is a surplus in the body. Drinking urine causes more of these substances to enter the body than normal. The body reacts to this by washing them away with water and other substances.

By ingesting urine, one stimulates the body not only to excrete part of these metabolic products at an accelerated rate, but also to convert another part into useful substances. A previously mentioned example of this is urea, which is converted through ammonia into glutamine.

Another consequence might be that substances which should normally leave the body with the urine, but have got stuck somewhere, now do so due to the accelerated flow. For example, in the case of gout, the body disposes of uric acid embedded in the joints.

The effects of flowing and cleansing are particularly noticeable while one is fasting. The first time one urinates while fasting, the urine is often thick and tastes strong, especially if one has a fever or is otherwise sick. However, after drinking this initial amount, the second flow of urine is thinner, even if one has not drunk extra water.

The re-use of urine, without ingesting extra liquid, yields a large amount of clear and not unpleasant tasting urine in a short period of time. According to this hypothesis, this ultimately results in stimulated and cleansed kidneys, and a purified bloodstream. At the same time, the intestines, skin and exhalation process probably entirely take over the role of secreting the unusable metabolic products.

9. Transmutation theory

Most of the former hypotheses will also be valid from a strictly mechanistic point of view. The transmutation theory, though, needs a new, holistic paradigm which is based more on the dynamics of energies. [36]

In recent scientific research, a shift is visible from reductionism to holism. It is beyond the scope of this book to go into this matter. I nevertheless want to take the new paradigm fully into account here in trying to find explanations for the effectiveness of urine therapy.

Urine can be considered to contain an exact holographic picture of the body fluids and tissues. The biofeedback of this holographic information by re-ingesting the urine may well inform the energy system in a way which helps restoring a disturbed balance.

The medical doctor and urine therapist Abele cautiously discusses the possible effect of urine as holographic feedback:

"The question rises as to whether urine could possibly be considered to be a sort of liquid-hologram. Once the body has been made conscious of urine in an unconventional way (such as it being reintroduced into the body by intramuscular injection) the whole organism evaluates it and subsequently updates its own regulating mechanisms (at least in specific cases)." [37]

The theory of transmutation implies that the body is capable, through energetic exchange within the body itself, to transmute certain substances or molecules into other ones. 'Short-circuiting' the system by ingesting one's own secreted body fluids might stimulate the transmutational forces within and challenge the body to transform unusable substances into usable ones without being constantly disturbed by new external input. This would specifically apply to fasting on urine.[38]

Another important aspect is the theory of structured water. The body consists for the biggest part of water and so does urine. Not all water is the same though. The molecular structure of water can be less or more organized and in the latter case one speaks of structured water. The more it is organized, the better all kind of enzymatic processes can do their job. These enzymatic processes, in their turn, are responsible and necessary for the digestion, absorption and transmutation of all nutrients.[39]

It is scientifically proven how water in biological systems becomes more organized. Water also becomes more organized through exposure to sunlight and through close contact with crystals. The body is both a receptor of sunlight and it contains a high amount of solid and liquid crystalline-like substances. Also body fluids themselves form fluid crystals.[40] Urine is thus a crystalline-like substance containing a high amount of structured water. This structured water, when taken in again, promotes better enzymatic functioning and it has a higher solubility for minerals. A higher amount of structured water in the body system is correlated with better health and more energy.[41]

The fact that urine is a liquid crystal substance, particularly because of the various salts in it, implies that it contains crystalline vibrations completely in tune with the vibrational condition of the body. Re-ingestion might give the body valuable vibrational information needed for two things. Healthy vibrations will strengthen the already existing, healthy body resonance. 'Diseased' or stress-vibrations will counteract any unhealthy resonance in the body. It is known that disturbing sounds of any sort can be counteracted best by confronting it with the same sounds.

The vibratory patterns of the body, both in the bones (solid crystals) and in the tissues and fluids (liquid crystals), play an important role in the process of transmutation. The resonance field of a crystal can make a protein, for example, change its form into one that is more useful for the body, or easier adaptable by it.[42]

Seeing urine as a liquid crystalline-like substance containing a high amount of structured water may help understanding its healing qualities on the more subtle levels.

10. Psychological effect

The shock initially brought on by drinking urine might fundamentally challenge previously accepted ideas, as a result of which repressed energy is released that can be applied to strengthen the body and fight an illness.

Scientists claim that the highest acceptable placebo effect is 30% (see section *5.1*). However, a much higher percentage of people actually achieves positive results with urine therapy, which is remarkable since many people are often initially skeptical because of their aversion to urine, and apply urine therapy as a last resort.

Confronting and conquering reluctance play an important role in this theory. Applying your own bodily substances in an attempt to heal can lead to a considerably broadened outlook on the intelligence and power of the body, and can increase your appreciation and love for yourself as a physical and spiritual being. Instead of regarding excretions (really just a part of yourself) as enemies, you regard them as your helpers. This healthier way of seeing yourself might well have a powerful healing effect on your body.

If the results are experienced as positive, applying your own urine as medication means that you have more physical and mental freedom than previously believed, which can also have a healing effect on a deep level.

Besides being beneficial on a personal level, the use of urine as medication opens a new door for contemporary medical science. It confronts us with the possibility that the powers of the body and the universe are infinite, and that we are much less dependent on complicated theories and technologies for our health than up until now was assumed.

Urine therapy confronts us with a very concrete 'healer within' which works both on a mechanistic and on an energetic level. The latter implies that urine, as a holographic substance, can affect all levels of being, from the physical, through the electromagnetic fields of the emotions and the mind, up to the subtler genetic vibrational information of the soul.

5.3 Some Individual Substances Found in Urine

We have discussed several hypotheses which might explain why urine therapy is effective. Several references were made to the many individual substances found in urine, including urea, which could positively affect a healing process. A general overview and a specified summary of a number of important substances usually found in urine follow below. The substances given in the specified summary have been researched, either in relation to urine therapy or in other contexts.

General Overview
(from recent Ciba-Geigy lists as presented in Dr.med. U.E. Hasler's book *Die Apotheke in uns*, see bibliography)

Anorganic substances in urine:
bicarbonate, chloride, phosphor, sulphur, bromide, fluoride, jodide, rhodanide, kalium, natrium, calcium, magnesium, iron, copper, zinc, cobalt, selenium, arsenium, lead, mercury.

Nitrogen-containing substances in urine:
nitrogen (as totality), urea, creatine, creatinine, guanidine, choline, carnitine, piperidine, spermi-dine, spermine, dopamine, adrenaline, nor-adrenaline, serotonin, tryptamine, amino-levulinic acid, porphyrin, bilirubin, and others.

Amino acids in urine:
alanine, carnosine, glycine, histidine, leucine, lysine, methionine, phenylalanine, serine, tyrosine, valine, hydroxyproline, galactosylhydroxylysine, xylo-sylserine, and others.

Proteins in urine:
albumin, haptoglobin, transferrin, IgG, IgA, IgM, and others.

Enzymes in urine:
lactatdehydrogenase, gamma-glutamyltransferase, alpha-amylase, uropepsinogen, lysozyme, beta-N-acetylglucosaminidase, urokinase, protease, and others.

Carbohydrates in urine:
arabinose, xylose, ribose, fucose, rhamnose, ketopentose, glucose, galactose, mannose, fructose, lactose, saccharose, fucosylglucose, raffinose, and others.

Nitrogen-free substances in urine:
wide range of organic acids

Vitamins in urine:
thiamine (vitamin B1), riboflavin (vitamin B2), vitamin B6, 4-pyridoxic acid, nicotinic acid, vitamin B-12, biopterine, ascorbic acid, and others.

Hormones in urine:
gonadotropin, corticotropin, prolactin, lactogenic hormones, oxytocin, vasopressin, thyroxine, cathe-cholamin (adrenaline, noradrenaline, dopamine), insulin, erythropoietin, corticosteroids (aldosterone, corticosterone, cortisone), testosterone, progesterone, oestrogen, and others.

Specified Summary

Agglutinins and precipitins – have a neutralizing effect on polio and other viruses.[43]

Antineoplaston – prevents selectively the growth of cancer cells without harming the growth of healthy cells.[44]

Allantoin – a nitrogenous crystal substance which helps heal wounds. It is an oxidation product of uric acid. This substance can be found in many skin cream products.[45]

DHEA (dehydroepiandrosterone or dehydroiso-androsterone) – a steroid secreted by the adrenal gland which can be found in large amounts in male urine. This substance prevents obesity, prolongs the lifespan of animals, and offers a possible treatment for anemia, diabetes and breast cancer in women. DHEA stimulates the growth of bone marrow and increases the production of substances manufactured by bone marrow such as red blood cells, monocytes, macrophages and lymphocytes. A low DHEA level seems to be linked to aging.[46]

'Gastric secretory depressants' – combat the growth of stomach ulcers.[47]

Glucuronic acid – is created in the liver, kidneys and intestinal canal and has an important secretion function.[48]

H-11 – inhibits the growth of cancer cells and reduces already existing tumors, without disturbing the recovery process.[49]

HUD (Human's Urine Derivative) – urine derivative shown to have remarkable anti-cancer properties.[50]

Interleukin-1 – this substance has a positive influence on helper cells and inhibiting substances. It can signal the hypothalamus to produce a fever.[51]

3-Methyl-glyoxal – destroys cancer cells, see also *Chapter 2.3*.[52]

Prostaglandin – is an hormonal substance which dilates the blood vessels and lowers blood pressure, relaxes the bronchial muscles, stimulates labor contractions, and has a number of other functions relating to the metabolism.[53]

Protein globulins – contain antibodies against specific allergens; identical to proteins in the immunoglobulins of serum (blood).[54]

Proteoses – immunologically active products of allergic reactions.[55]

Retine – anti-cancer element extracted from urine.[56]

Urea – see *Chapter 5.2*, section *5. Re-absorption of urea*.[57]

Urine peptide (or polypeptide) – shows tuberculo-static activity which has been isolated in chemically pure form.[58]

Uric acid – helps keep 'free radical scavengers' (molecules which can cause cancer) under control, combats old age, and even has a tuberculostatic effect.[59]

Urokinase – see *Chapter 5.2*, section *3*. *Re-absorption of enzymes.*[60]

5.4   References

1. B. Bartnett, p. 10, see *Bibliography*.
2. A.H. Free & H.M. Free,*'Nature and Composition of Urine from Healthy Subjects'*, in Urinalysis in Clinical Laboratory Practice, CRC Press, Cleveland, Ohio, 1975, pp. 13 & 17.
3. B. Bartnett, p. 10, see *Bibliography*; J. Plesch, *'Urine therapy'*, Medical Press (London), vol. 218, August 6, 1947, pp. 128-133.
4. *'Immuno-Tolerance: Historical Perspective'*, Physicians Handbook, 1982, p. 13.
5. C.H. Duncan, *'Gonorrhea: Its Prevention and Cure by Autotherapy'*, Medical Record; March 30, 1912, p. 610; idem, *'Autotherapy'*, New York Medical Journal, December 21, 1912, p. 1281.
6. Dr. William D. Linscott, *'Specific Immunologic Unresponsiveness'*, 3rd edition of Basic & Clinical Immunology, a Lange Medical Publication, Los Altos, California, Chapter 17, 'Historical Perspective', Physician's Handbook, 1982.
7. J. Wynhausen, *'Urea: Its Possible Role in Auto-Urine Therapy'*, in Shivambu Kalpa Parishad, compilation, Goa India 1993; Martha M. Christy, Your Own Perfect Medicine, see *Bibliography*.
8. S.S. Saraswati, see *Bibliography*, p. 31-32.
9. J. Wynhausen, see above, note 7.
10. See also Professor Jean Rostand's comment as reproduced in Chapter 2.3 of this book.
11. M. Mills & T. Faunce, *'Melatonin Supplementation from Early Morning Auto-Urine Drinking'*, Medical Hypotheses, vol. 36, p. 195; G. Vines, New Scientist 29, February 1992, p. 20.
12. Lissoni et al., Oncology, 1991; 48(6):448-50.
13. B.F. John, see *Bibliography*.
14. Staff Reporter, *'Now Urine Business'*, Hippocrates (magazine), May 1988; Tierärztliche Umschau, 4/1984; M. Duffy et al., *'Urokinase-Plasminogen Activator, A Marker for Aggressive Breast Carcinomas'*, Cancer, vol. 62, no. 3, August 1, 1988, pp. 531-533; Staff Writers, *'Blood Clots: Legs and Lungs'*, Harvard Medical School Health Letter, vol. 10, no. 3, January 1985, p. 5.
15. J. Wynhausen, see above, note 7.
16. D.J. Pochopien, *'Urea and Glucose Concentrations of Amniotic Fluid during Pregnancy. Amniotic Fluid: Research and Clinical Application'*, D.V.I. Fairweather & T.K.A.B. Eskes (editors), Excerpta Medica, Amsterdam 1973.
17. G. Kolata, *'Surgery on Foetuses Reveals They Heal Without Scars'*, New York Times, August 16, 1988, p. C1 & C3.
18. Walsery Mackenzie & Bodenlos, *'Urea Metabolism in Man'*, Journal of Clinical Investigation 38 (1959), p. 1617.
19. Haussinger, Deiter & Sies, Glutamine Metabolism in Mammalian Tissues, Springer Verlag, New York 1984.
20. R. Peat, *'Sharks, Salmon and Osmotic Therapies'*, Townsend Letter for Doctors, July 1991.
21. A. Ackerson & C. Resnick, *'The Effects of L-*

Glutamine, N-Acetyl-D-Glucosamine, Gamma-Linolenic Acid and Gamma-Oryzanol on Intestinal Permeability', Townsend Letter for Doctors, January 1993.

22. Haussinger, etc., see above, note 19.

23. M. Javid, 'Urea in Intracranial Surgery', Journal of Neurosurgery, 1961, vol. 18, nr. 1, p. 51-57; id., 'Effect of Urea on Cerebrospinal Fluid Pressure in Human Subjects', Journal of the American Medical Association, 1956.

24. M. Murayama & R.M. Nalbandian, Sickle Cell Hemoglobin: Molecule to Man, Little Brown, Boston 1973.

25. E.D. Danopoulos, article in The Lancet, January 26, 1974; E.D. Danopoulos & M. Wayne, 'Progress in Treating Malignancies with Urea and in Combination with Creatine Hydrate', Townsend Letter for Doctors, December 1990.

26. R.J. Feldman & H.I. Maibach, 'Percutaneous Penetration of Hydrocortisone with Urea', Archives of Dermatology 109, p. 58-59; Gunnar Swanbeck, 'Urea in the Treatment of Dry Skin', Department of Dermatology, Göteborg Sweden, 1992; Jorgen Serup, 'A Double-Blind Comparison of Two Creams containing Urea as the Active Ingredient', University of Copenhagen, Denmark, Acta Derm Venereol, 1992.

27. J.U. Schlegel et al., 'Bactericidal Effect of Urea', Journal of Urology, vol. 86, no. 6, December 1961, pp. 819-822; E. Bello, 'The Original Therapy of Wounds with Urine, Practice Traditional with Peruvian Indians, Explained and Justified', Revista Medica de Vera Cruz (Mexico), vol. 20, no. 4, April 1, 1940, pp. 3067-3071.; H.W. Smith 'De Urina', Journal of the American Medical Association, vol. 155, no. 10, July 3, 1954, pp. 899-902.

28. K.B. Bjornesjo, 'On the Effect of Human Urine on Tubercle Bacilli: II The Tuberculostatic Effect of Various Urine Constituents', Acta Scandinavica, vol. 25, no. 5, 1951, pp. 447-455; Q. Myrvik et al., 'Studies on the Tuberculoinhibitory Properties of Ascorbic Acid Derivatives and Their Possible Role in Inhibition of Tubercle Bacilli by Urine', American Review of Tuberculosis, vol. 69, no. 3, March, 1954, pp. 406-418; Shusuke Tsuji et al., 'Isolation from Human Urine of A Polypeptide Having Marked Tuberculostatic Activity', Fifth Division of the Tuberculosis Research Institute, Kyoto University, Japan 1965.

29. 'Immuno-Tolerance: Historical Perspective', Physician's Handbook, 1982, p. 7.

30. Carmelo Giordano, 'Use of Exogenous and Endogenous Urea for Protein Synthesis in Normal and Uremic Subjects', Naples University School of Medicine, 1963.

31. C.W.M. Wilson & A. Lewis, 'Auto-Immune Therapy Against Human Allergic Disease: A Physiological Self Defense Factor', Medical Hypothesis, vol. 12, 1983, p. 143-158; C.H. Duncan, 'Autotherapy', New York Medical Journal, December 21, 1912; M.W. Turner & D.S. Rowe, 'Antibodies of IgA and IgC Class in Normal Human Urine', Immunology, vol. 12, 1967, p. 689; Nancy Dunne, 'The Use of Injected and Sublingual Urine in the Treatment of Allergies', Oxford Medical Symposium, 1981.

32. Herz/Abele, p. 26, see Bibliography; Dr. R. Tiberi, 'Auto-Urine Vaccine Therapy for Acute Hemorrhagic Nephritis', Institute of Clinical Medicine, University of Perugia, Italy 1934.

33. Herz/Abele, p. 27, see Bibliography; Excerpts from the 7th Conference on AIDS/3rd STD World Congress, Amsterdam 1992 (pob 3621, poc 4494, poc 4430, poc 4447, poc 4764, thc

1582)

34. R. Peat, see above, note 20; Eaton M. MacKay & Charles R. Schroeder, *'Virucidal (Rabies and Poliomyelitis) Activity of Aqeous Urea Solutions'*, American Proceedings of the Society of Experimental Biology 35, pp. 74-76, 1936; Leon Muldavis & Jean M. Holtzman, *'Treatment of Infected wounds with Urea'*, The London Lancet, 1938; John H. Foulger, M.D., *'The Action of Urea and Some of Its Derivatives on Bacteria'* & *'The Antiseptic and Bacterial Action of Urea'*, Journal of Laboratory and Clinical Medicine, University of Cincinatti, 1935; Donald Kaye, *'Antibacterial Activity of Human Urine'*, Cornell University Medical College, 1968; Robert C. Noble, M.D. & M. Parekh, *'Bactericidal Properties of Urine for Neisseria Gonorrhea'*, Journal of Sexually Transmitted Diseases, 1987

35. Herz/Abele, p. 26, see *Bibliography*.

36. See e.g. Richard Gerber, M.D., Vibrational Medicine, Bear & Company, Santa Fe NM 1988.

37. Herz/Abele, p. 27, see *Bibliography*.

38. See specifically the chapter on urine therapy and alchemy in Dr. Schaller's Amaroli, see *Bibliography*.

39. Gabriel Cousens, M.D., Spiritual Nutrition and the Rainbow Diet, Cassandra Press, San Rafael CA 1986, p. 22; Friedman, H.L., Krishman, C.V. and Jolicoeur, C., *'Ionic Interactions in Water'*, Ann. N.Y. Academic of Science 1972, 204: pp. 77-99; Clegg, James, *'Metabolism and the Intracellular Environment: The Vicinal Water Network Model'*, in Cell Associated Water, (Drost-Hansen, W. and James Clegg; eds.) New York: Academic Press, 1979, pp. 363-413.

40. Cousens, see note 39 above, p. 89-96; Lipton, Bruce, *'Liquid Crystal Consciousness, The Cellular Basis of Life'*, presented at First International Crystal Conference, San Francisco CA 1986.

41. Cousens, see note 39 above, p. 23; Mikesell, N., *'Cellular Rgeneration'*, Psychic Research Newsletter, San Jose 1985, pp. 1-10.

42. Lipton, Bruce, see note 40.

43. A.M. Lerner et al., *'Neutralizing Antibody to Polioviruses in Normal Human Urine'*, Journal of Clinical Investigation, vol. 41, no. 4, April 1962, pp. 805-815; L.A. Hanson et al., *'Characterization of Antibodies in Human Urine'*, Journal of Clinical Investigation, vol. 44, no. 5, 1965, pp. 703-715; J. Plesch, *'Urine therapy'*, Medical Press (London), vol. 218, August 6, 1947, pp. 128-133.

44. G.J.W. Ollerenshaw, *'Observations on Dosage of H-11 Extract'*, Medical World, London, vol. 64, March 1, 1946, pp. 72-76; S.R. Burzynski et al., *'Antineoplaston A in Cancer Therapy'*, Physiology, Chemistry & Physics, vol. 9, 1977, p. 485; Staff Reporter, *'Antineoplastons: New Antitumor Agents Stil High Expectations'*, Oncology News, vol. 16, no. 4, July-August 1990, p. 1.

45. Bartnett, p. 8; Allmann, p. 121, see *Bibliography*.

46. S. Kent, *'DHEA: Miracle Drug?'*, Geriatrics, vol. 37, no. 9, 1982, pp. 157-161; J.S. James, *'DHEA: Mystery AIDS Treatment'*, Aids Treatment News, Issue 48, January 1, 1988, pp. 1-6.

47. D.J. Sandweiss et al., *'The Effect of Urine Extracts on Peptic Ulcers'*, American Journal of Digestive Diseases, vol. 8, no. 10, October, 1941, pp. 371-382.

48. Allmann, p. 121, see bibliography.
49. H.H. Thompson, *'H-11 for Cancer'*, British Medical Journal, July 31, 1943, p. 149; G.J.W. Ollerenshaw, *'Observations on Dosage of H-11 Extract'*, Medical World, London, vol. 64, March 1, 1946, pp. 72-76.
50. Momoe Soda, *'Treatment of Gastric Cancer with HUD, an Antigenic Substance Obtained from Patient's Urine'*, Tokyo 1968.
51. E. Kimball et al., *'Interleukin-1 Activity in Normal Human Urine'*, source and date unknown; Z. Liao et al., *'Identification of a Specific Interleukin-1 Inhibitor in the Urine of Febrile patients'*, Journal of Experimental Medicine, Rockefeller University Press, vol. 159, January, 1984, pp. 126-136.
52. Allmann, p. 122, see *Bibliography*.
53. Bartnett, p. 9; Allmann, p. 123, see *Biblio graphy*.
54. T. Tomasi et al., *'Characteristics of an Immune System Common to Certain External Secretions'*, Journal of Experimental Medicine, vol. 121, no. 1, January, 1965, pp. 101-122; C.H. Duncan, *'Autotherapy'*, New York Medical Journal, December 21, 1912, pp. 1278-1283.
55. W. Darley et al., *'Studies on Urinary Proteose; Skin Reactions and Therapeutic Applications in Hay Fever'*, Annals of Internal Medicine, vol. 6, no. 3, 1932, pp. 389-399.
56. Albert Szent-Gyorgi et al., *'Preparation of Retine from Human Urine'*, Science Magazine 1963.
57. G. Decaux et al., *'5-Year Treatment of the Chronic Syndrome of Inappropriate Secretion of ADH with Oral Urea'*, Department of Internal Medicine, Erasmus University Hospital, Belgium 1993.
58. K.B. Bjornesjo, *'Tuberculostatic Factor in Normal Human Urine'*, American Review of Tuberculosis, vol. 73, no. 6, June, 1956, p. 967; S. Tsuji et al., *'Isolation from Human Urine of a Polypeptide Having Marked Tuberculostatic Activity'*, American Review of Respiratory Diseases, vol. 91, no. 6, June, 1965, pp. 832-838.
59. Davies Owens, *'Youthful Uric Acid'*, Omni, October, 1982; K.B. Bjornesjo, *'On the Effect of Human Urine on Tubercle Bacilli: II The Tuberculostatic Effect of Various Urine Constituents'*, Acta Scandinavica, vol. 25, no. 5, 1951, pp. 447-455.
60. P.M. Mannuci & A. D'Angelo, Urokinase, Basic and Clinical Aspects, 1982.

6. A SOURCE OF INSPIRATION:
Personal Experiences with Urine Therapy

This chapter gives an overview of various personal experiences from people who have worked with urine therapy. The number of stories which follow is limited, and some have been borrowed from other literature on urine therapy. An abundance of reports and experiences can be found in other books on urine therapy, the titles of which are listed in the bibliography.

This chapter also contains a number of reports from urine therapists with whom I have spoken or corresponded. These letters and reports give an impression of the objective and personal experiences of those who professionally work with urine therapy. They provide a lively illustration to my own story about my introduction to, experiences with and research on urine therapy. Personal stories were the inspiring factor in my journey. I hope to pass along some of this inspiration in this way.

6.1 Reports from Urine Therapists

Letter from Dr. Chandrika Prasad Mishra
Shastri "Ayurved-Ratna"
Auto-Urine Specialist
Adanpur, India   28 December 1992

Many thanks for your letter dated 4 November. Unfortunately, I could not reply earlier due to political disturbances and curfew impositions from 6-24 December.

To introduce my humble self, it is sufficient to mention that I: (1) am presently 86 years old and in sound health, (2) was originally (since 1929) a staunch freedom fighter in the non-cooperation movement of Mahatma Gandhi, and (3) have been serving humanity at large for the past 32 years with auto-urine-therapy (Shivambu Kalpa). I have been publishing a bi-weekly journal called *Shivambu Mitra* since 1980 and preach urine therapy throughout the country.

By the grace of God Almighty and with the blessings and good wishes of associates, collaborators, colleagues and sincere friends like yourself, together with the unique strength of this God-gifted nectar (Shivambu), I have successfully cured or eradicated numerous illnesses, acute as well as chronic, without any difficulty. These include illnesses such as asthma, diabetes, gout (rheumatism), high blood pressure, etc., in addition to various common and dreaded diseases such as cancer, AIDS, heart ailments, etc.

The time has come for all of us to meet and join hands to spread this sacred mission of health consciousness, health education and health services throughout the world, so that the World Health Organization (W.H.O.) will be persuaded to include urine therapy among other medical treatments, the most of which are failing, falling, deteriorating or fading away.

With this enthusiasm, we are going to hold an All India Conference on Urine Therapy (Shivambu Kalpa) in Goa in 1993.

Please do not hesitate to write me about your present health, happiness and financial position. Also, please state your age, height, weight, education, experience, business or vocation, family circumstances, etc. so I can map out a fruitful future for your ambitions.

In the meantime, I enclose a copy of an article published in Taipeh dated October 8, 1992 which also proves the popularity of urine therapy in Taiwan.

Thank you once again.

Affectionately yours,

Dr. Chandrika Prasad Mishra

Letter from Balkrishna Laxman Nalavade
Auto-Urine Consultant
Poona, India   5 December 1992

'Om, All Life Is One'

I was very glad to receive your letter dated 4 November. As I was out of town for a few weeks, I apologize for my delayed reply.

I started practicing urine therapy in 1969 after miraculously curing myself of a variety of diseases. From the age of 25 to 40, my body was, as it were, a 'museum' of diseases, namely stomach-ache, amoebic dysentery, constipation, appendicitis, piles, kidney stones, neurosis, backache, heart weakness, etc. No therapy could cure me completely.

A renowned physician examined me in 1968 and declared that I only had a few months to live! However, due to God's providence, I was completely cured by urine therapy within approximately two and a half months. After this miracle cure, I started practicing this therapy in Poona, my home since 1969.

Thousands of patients suffering from various fatal and chronic diseases and abandoned by allopathic doctors have been cured by urine therapy. Among the various natural methods of treatment, urine therapy is the most simple, effective and safe, and it is universally available 24 hours a day. For even better results, urine therapy can safely be combined with acupressure, acupuncture, yoga, spiritual healing, tele-therapy, herbal medicines, colour therapy, homoeopathy, prayers, meditations, etc. Urine therapy is the gift of God – a panacea – for human beings and animals.

For further information, I enclose a copy of my paper which I read at the World Congress of Natural Medicines. I am very happy to hear that you practice this very useful therapy.

Since 1969 my life has been a 'bonus life', leased to me by His Almighty, which I have been using for the propagation of urine therapy to aid suffering humanity.

Since December is the festival and holy month, we (myself and my family members) wish you, your family members and friends a Happy Christmas and New Year.

May God bless you all with a long, happy, healthy and creative life.

If you happen to visit India, please do come to stay in our home in Poona and give us the chance to act as your host.

With kind regards,

Yours sincerely,

B.L. Nalavade

Letter from D. Satyamurthy
Employee Bethany Colony
Bapatla, India   27 December 1992

I am a paramedic worker at Bethany Colony where people with leprosy are treated. I was told of this treatment by a woman from England, Sister Margaret Deleney. Together, we treated several leprosy topical ulcers and some chronic asthma cases and skin disorders. We achieved good results with this treatment. Since then, I have treated many cases, and the treatment has never failed. Also, hip baths and drinking urine daily is the best treatment for chronic and painful piles. The problem is that the patient is often unwilling to drink his or her own water. Therefore we mix it with some juice and serve it at breakfast.

I can honestly say it is the best treatment for leprosy ulcers, asthma and several skin disorders. I am extremely grateful for this therapy and plan to start a small clinic for urine therapy.

D. Satyamurthy

Declaration from Dr. Jagdip Shah, renowned doctor in Bombay and speaker at the First All India Conference On Urine Therapy, India 1993.

I am a gynecologist, and started taking an interest in urine therapy after six years of clinical experience. During this period, I became aware of the limitations of allopathy. After having become acquainted with urine therapy and having received my Naturopathy Diploma, I started applying this knowledge in the treatment of several of my patients – not only gynecological and obstetric patients, but with other patients as well.

I was astonished by the results of this therapy on several diseases which allopathic science cannot treat, let alone cure. Within two years, I have treated the following diseases with a combination of urine therapy and dietary changes with astonishingly good results: herpes genitalis, prostatic enlargement (benign), multiple kidney stones, hypothyroidism, rheumatoid erosions and leucorrhoea, chronic sinusitis, allergic dermatitis, and many more.

Scientific base: Research conducted in many countries has proven the nutritional value of urine due to its high level of proteins, hormones, minerals, vitamins and other valuable substances. These are easily assimilated and recycled by the body without any loss of energy.

Urine contains immunologically active substances which fight viral and bacterial infections and boost the immunological potential even if one is immunologically weak, as is the case with AIDS, cancer, or any debilitating illness.

Urine is a powerful cleansing agent which detoxifies and eliminates all poisonous elements. Urine therapy combined with a fast and/or a diet of raw fruits and vegetables greatly helps eliminate these toxic substances from the body within a few weeks.

Urine has an anti-cancer activity – many substances have been isolated from urine which have been scientifically proven to be effective in preventing and reducing the growth of cancer.

Dr. P.D. Desai is of the opinion that the harm done to humanity by modern, potent drugs, vaccines, radiation and unnecessary surgery is far greater than the damage resulting from the atom bomb. The damage from the atom bomb is confined to the place where the atom bomb explodes and for a limited period of time, while the damage done by potent drugs, etc. is spread through every country of the world, throughout the year, day and night.

The following is a reaction from Stanislaw R. Burzynski, scientific researcher and discoverer of the anti-cancer substance Antineoplast, to the Urine Therapy Centre in Ahmedabad, India. He discusses the possible link between Antineoplast and the positive results of urine therapy as it is applied in India.

The main interest of our research are the compounds which we have named Antineoplast. They have very potent anticancer activity without causing any harm to the normal human tissues. In the last year we were able to treat successfully 14 different types of human cancers including bladder, colon, tongue, breast, lung, ovarian and uterine cancer – all of them with metastases to distant organs, even to the brain. The result of these studies are in press now. Antineo-plastons, which chemically are medium sized peptides, are produced by healthy human tissues and are present in blood and urine. At the present time we are isolating them from normal human urine. The concentration of Antineoplastons in urine is very small and usually it is necessary to process 29 gallons of urine to obtain a daily dose for one patient. This amount of the medication is dissolved in a very small volume and given the same way as Insulin injections. We were able to have complete remission in four to six weeks in medium advanced cases. At the present time we do not see any adverse reaction. It is my great pleasure to know that in India you have good results with auto-uro-therapy, because it may support our theory. Western medicine took a lot from Indian folk medicine. We are glad to know that our therapy may have the links with natural treatment done for centuries.

(From: *Manav Mootra*, Raojibhai Patel, Ahmedabad 1991)

6.2 Some Personal Stories

Ms. W.M., The Netherlands

"I discovered urine therapy in India, where I lived for quite some time. I regularly came across a man at the bank where I did my banking. One day he did not show up, and I heard from others that he had typhoid, a serious, debilitating and often fatal illness. I regularly inquired after his health, and heard that with each attack it was expected that he would die. Some time later, however, I saw him at the bank again, and he was in the pink of health!

Only later did I hear from him how he had regained his health. I had told him that my own children were seriously ill, and he told me that he had cured himself of typhoid with urine therapy.

My four children all had a blood disease known as mononucleosis. They were weak, fatigued and listless, and constantly ran a fever. I had my two youngest children urinate into a brown bottle, and later gave this to them as medicine, without letting them know that they were drinking their own urine. My nanny was a great help – she even encouraged me to try this method. She came from Kerala, a state in the south of India where, as she told me, many fishermen also used urine. They often cut themselves on the fish, causing rather nasty infections, in which case urine can be used as an effective remedy. For a few days, I had my children fast and massaged them every day for a few hours with urine. At first it was difficult, as my husband was completely against this method. Some time later, I had my children repeat the fast for a period of ten days, and they responded positively. Their health greatly improved: they regained their healthy appetites, performed much better at school and were more creative. Apparently, they were cleansed on many inner levels.

Of course, I also decided to try urine therapy. Ever since I was eighteen, I had suffered from bronchitis, sinusitis, and chronic anemia. After trying urine therapy, I felt much better. Furthermore, the laboratory technicians were astonished at the sudden rise in my haemoglobin percentage, which had increased to the accepted standard!

I later stopped using urine therapy, until I discovered that I had a tumor in my breast which was likely to become malignant. Initially, nobody wanted to help and support me in treating the tumor with urine therapy. The alternatives were chemical medication and probably a breast amputation. I wanted to prevent this at all costs.

At that time, I met Elly, a Dutch woman living in an ashram in India. She supported me, and I went with my family to the ashram where I regularly drank my own urine. I decided not to constantly check and see if the tumor was still there, and at one point I discovered that it was gone. At that time, I had only drunk my urine, without massaging myself with it.

I also used urine to heal wounds. I treated somebody with third-degree burns with urine therapy, and practically no scars remained. I also successfully applied urine compresses when my children had scrapes or were bitten by jellyfish or insects.

I used to be a nurse, and know quite a bit about medicine. I worked in the operation room, in district nursing and in private nursing, and have seen allopathic medicine fail many times, which makes it easier for me to work with urine therapy. In India, I worked quite a lot with natural medicine. Whenever I heard about a therapy that helped improve health, I researched it and tried it out. In this way, I have become acquainted with a number of different therapies. But urine therapy beats them all! Nothing is better than urine therapy."

Ms. L.T., The Netherlands

"I am forty years old and work as a journalist. The first three months that I worked with urine therapy, I wrote a book, moved, and kept my routine going as a single working mother. This should give you an idea about the enormous amount of energy I possessed. At the time, there was also an influenza epidemic in the Netherlands and almost everybody I knew had been sick, myself excluded. One night it began, starting with a pounding, infected feeling in my nose and gums (a weak spot), a dry throat and teary eyes. I figured it was logical that I break down once the greatest pressure was over. I gargled and rinsed my gums with fresh urine and doubled the daily dose of urine I normally drank. A day and a half later, I was completely recovered, and did not even have a runny nose any more. The flu, or whatever it was, had not intensified.

In the initial phase, perhaps the most remarkable effect of urine was on my moods. Drinking my own urine helped me break down barriers I never thought I could, and gave me a delightful feeling of inner freedom. It was something like, 'If I can do this, I can do almost anything.' Like go to Australia, or whatever. That feeling of freedom has remained."

Mr. E.J.P., The Netherlands

"Around 1975 I heard and read about urine therapy for the first time. That was in Bombay, India.

Much earlier, when I was eleven years old, I had heard about and seen this remarkable ritual in which freshly discharged urine is consumed, for example by animals (goats and certain apes use this method during illness).

It certainly was interesting that this ancient, exceptional knowledge should once again enter my life in the form of a book by Acharya Jagdish B. He is an Indian publisher who had made it his mission in life to promote and popularize this excellent, personal therapy. In this same period, the Indian prime minister Morarji Desai made no bones about the fact that drinking urine was the secret of his virility and energetic attitude towards life. If I remember correctly, this man was well into his seventies and still functioned as prime minister. I recently heard that he is now in his nineties and still leads an active and healthy life.

Although I was familiar with this fantastic therapy and had heard that it can help cure illnesses such as cancer, leukemia, gangrene and many other infections, I could not bring myself to directly try out this method.

This happened approximately four years later. In all that time, I still had not found anybody who was experienced in this method, and so I had to rely on my feeling which told me that this knowledge was indeed valuable. Fate placed me in a situation in which I was put in an isolation cell for alleged dealing in hash while on vacation in Northern Europe. In order to get released from the isolation cell and into the hospital, where a friend of mine was hospitalized, I decided to see what would happen if I drank my own urine. If it made me sick, my experiment would be a success; if not, I would have to try something else in order to be taken to the hospital.

The first morning, I immediately spit out the first sip of urine before it even touched my tongue, and threw away the rest of the urine. Disgusting, I thought, I'll never do that again.

The next morning, motivated by my desire to get to the hospital as quickly as possible, I tried drinking my own urine for a second time, once again with the same unpleasant result; mental blocks can sometimes be obstinate barriers.

The third day, I finally succeeded in swallowing a full sip of urine. I sat quietly in order to analyze what might happen. The taste was not as bad as I had expected – a lightly salty aftertaste which disappeared rather quickly. Incidentally, I have drunk more disgusting tasting liquids prescribed by the doctor in order to improve my health.

Approximately five minutes later, I quite urgently had to defecate. No sooner had I sat on the toilet than I defecated quickly and easily, which was remarkable since I had been suffering from constipation from the unhealthy prison food. Five minutes later I defecated again, and finally felt relieved.

Since that morning, I have repeated this ritual every day and have not suffered from constipation. Remarkably enough, a dozen small warts which I had had my whole life on my hands also disappeared after eight days, as if they had suddenly fallen off. A few pustules arose here and there, one of which burst open after a ripening process of approximately eight days, releasing one and a half teaspoons of pus. Obviously, a

cleansing process had started in my body. After a number of weeks in which I ritually drank my morning urine, I noticed that changes were slowly beginning to take place in my body. Now, after using urine for fourteen years, I can confirm that I am 99% less susceptible to all kinds of epidemics, flus, infections and other miseries to which I used to be very susceptible. You do not have to be sick in order to start urine therapy. In theory, urine therapy increases your resistance to illness, and sometimes small irregularities come to the surface and can be dealt with.

I hope this story sheds more light on the positive effects of urine therapy and wish every researcher success with his or her research and findings with this 'ultimate survival' method."

Ms. M.v.L., The Netherlands

"In my opinion, Shivambu Kalpa (urine therapy) is the most miraculous and effective way to treat all physical ailments and illnesses. The best thing about this therapy is that it not only eliminates the symptoms, but also works on the causes. That's how I see it: truth, simplicity and love.

I was first introduced to this therapy approximately twelve years ago. In the Babaji's ashram in India where I was staying, I came across an Australian man standing on a ladder, painting the temple walkway. His feet were on eye level, and I could see that they were covered with wounds and sores. I called to him, "Hey John, you've got to do something about those feet of yours." He answered, "Yes, yes, I piss on them." I said to him, motherly as I am, "Come on, John, don't be angry, I have some powerful calendula ointment." He answered once again, "No, no, I simply piss on them."

After calling back and forth to each other, he came down from the ladder and explained his therapy to me. I did not believe a word of what he said, and kept going on about my calendula ointment. "There is a book in the library you should read," he said. I was completely baffled when I read it, but I felt, I knew it was good.

After a week, his feet were as clean and smooth as a baby's bottom. I used urine when I had a sore throat and for small scrapes, and started to tell people about urine therapy. Later, however, I more or less forgot about it and started using other medication again. A few years later, I hiked through the jungle in the 'wrong' shoes, as I had lost my good shoes. When I got home, my right foot looked terrible – the big toe was completely open and full of dirt. I tried calendula. The second day, my foot was terribly swollen and was very painful. The local doctor said that I either had to take antibiotics or my foot would have to be amputated. I suddenly remembered John and his wonder drug. I placed a cloth soaked in my own urine on my toes and foot, up to the ankle, and wrapped a plastic bag around the cloth. I was a sight! But I knew it would work. Within a few hours, the pain was gone, although the wounds on my toes and the swelling were still there. The doctor panicked and became angry with me. But I did not want to take antibiotics. The first two days, I changed the urine cloths every two hours and drank the rest of the urine. Within a week, my foot was better. The doctor was still angry, but surprised as well. I gave him Armstrong's book on urine therapy. Actually, he was already familiar with the therapy, but as an Indian doctor he thought working with antibiotics was 'more impressive'. Since then, this doctor has cured many people with Shivambu Kalpa (urine therapy).

In the last ten years, I have worked a great deal with urine therapy and have achieved spectacular results.

Earaches, eye infections, fever, burns (also sunburn): urine therapy has helped heal all of these ailments. It changed the life of a German girl, whom I met in India. Whenever the temperature rose even just a little, she would be covered with eczema. I once asked her, "Why do you always wear long-sleeve shirts and long skirts when it is so hot?" She rolled up her sleeve and said, "That's why." A terrible case of eczema covered the skin on her arms and legs. Following my advice, she started to rub her own urine onto her arms and legs. The pain and itching disappeared immediately, and after a few days, her arms were only red. She plucked up the courage to drink urine, and gained so much faith in her healing that she even started drinking extra water so that she would produce more urine. After two weeks, the eczema had completely disappeared. And it has not come back since!

Urine therapy has convinced me of the healing power we all possess within ourselves, not only metaphysical but also physical. Thank you, my body, for the magical power of your water. I bow in respect for *the water of life*!"

Mr. V.M., Germany

"I'll say it straight off: I do not have any great, miraculous recovery to report. When I was a child, I tasted my urine out of curiosity. It tasted sharp and burned a bit, and I could not imagine that I would ever drink it again.

Nevertheless, I heard from a good friend about the positive effects of urine, and after a long period of doubt, I tried it anyway. I woke up one day and knew right away that today would be the day. So I urinated into a glass, smelled it and emptied the glass in one draught. I was amazed. It tasted and smelled neutral.

The only thing I found to be unpleasant was the temperature. The following morning, I decided to drink another glass of urine; however, the smell made me dump the urine immediately in the toilet.

Only some time later did I consider drinking urine once again – I had diarrhea, my partner had left me and I felt generally weak. The situation could not get much worse, and so I drank my own fresh urine the whole day. After only two or three glasses, I felt less exhausted and from that moment on, things started improving.

Whenever I had trouble drinking urine because of the taste, I held my nose, drank the urine and rinsed with water. Since then, I drink my urine every day and massage my whole body with it. My dry skin is not flaky any more, and I do not have to go through life with skin cream, which was impossible before I started using urine. Furthermore, urine leaves skin with a pleasant, slightly sweet, warm scent.

It is interesting to perform a 'urine-test' every morning regarding the colour, smell, taste and substance. In this way, you can learn more about your body, feelings, food, etc. It is also exciting to hear new stories about this 'unusual liquid' and to try out new recipes.

For example, when I heard that, long before Christ, people used urine to do the laundry and keep the house clean, I tried an experiment myself. I mixed fresh urine with urine that was approximately 1/22 year old (it smelled like pure ammonia) and used this mixture to wash the windows. It not only dissolved the dirt on the windows, but also the paint spots and a number of other spots which I had not been able to clean with any other cleanser. The same thing happened when I cleaned a mirror with old urine. Moreover, it did not smell dirty, my hands were smooth, I could water the plants with the cleaning water without a guilty conscience, and my windows were perfectly clean!

Because I have never been seriously ill, I unfortunately do not have any spectacular recoveries to report, at least not from myself. Even so, I strongly believe that urine therapy is good. This is why I continue to use urine."

Ms. H.P., The Netherlands

"I have suffered from rheumatism for years, especially in my hands. My son told me about urine therapy and suggested I use urine compresses. This surprised me, but I started treating my hands daily with urine. The result was extraordinary. Besides the fact that my hands felt much smoother, the most remarkable thing was that the pain practically disappeared."

Ms. A.O., The Netherlands

"My hair was dried out due to a perm and coloring. After rubbing four-day-old urine into my hair and letting it soak in overnight, I noticed that it had become softer and more manageable. I also massaged myself with fresh urine for a week, and then started drinking it with orange juice. The first few days, I felt quite healthy, but subsequently began to feel less fit. My sleeping pattern changed – I sometimes needed a lot of sleep, sometimes very little. I also felt depressed from time to time. I see this as a purification process."

Ms. D.V., The Netherlands

"I would like to tell you about my experiences with urine therapy. I am 60 years old, have three children and am convinced that the cures for many illnesses are often simple and obvious.

For more than a year, I had been suffering from an allergic reaction to cosmetics and often had a terrible rash. I repressed the rash with hormonal ointment. Last summer, I stopped using the ointment and tried urine therapy.

1 August: I started drinking my own urine (at first with an aversion, but I quickly got used to it). I drank almost all of my day- and night-urine and rubbed it into my arms as well. (Urine has such a beautiful colour!) After swimming, I rubbed urine all over my body. Result: my dried out skin covered with rashes became soft and smooth.

7 August: The rash began to change: spots disappeared, and returned; the rash started to burn more, then less. I started rubbing four-day-old urine into my skin (it stank!). The skin on my hands, which was old and wrinkly, became soft and smooth.

10 August: For months, one of my teeth hurt whenever I drank cold water. The pain was now gone!

For a year, I had suffered from dizziness due to an inner ear infection. This condition improved considerably. Every day, I rubbed urine into my skin and hair, which became soft and shiny. I was less stressed out and had a powerful feeling of inner peace.

13 August: The rash did not disappear quickly enough for me, so I placed a compress of old urine on my arms and covered it with plastic. The next morning, the rash was gone! I could not believe my eyes. Over the course of the day, the rash returned and started to burn again and my day urine also tasted bitter. I stopped swimming and wrapped the compresses around my arms every evening. Every morning, the spots looked better.

17 August: I was nauseous at night and the following morning. I also felt diarrhea coming on and was terribly tired. I stayed in bed, slept a lot, drank extra (herbal) tea and did not eat. I had a bit of diarrhea and the nausea was gone. From this point on, I drank my urine three times a day, covered my arms in the evening with urine compresses and washed myself in the morning with urine. Besides the spots, my skin looked terrific. I noticed that I sometimes breathed deeply, a cross between a sigh and a gasp. This felt like a kind of release, as if everything was falling into place. I also cut salt out of my diet.

19 August: After six days of compresses, the rash was almost gone! I did it without the use of hormonal ointment. My entire system was more in balance, and I suspected that this would influence my total development (physical and spiritual). It is incredible that our bodies produce a medicine, always at our disposal.

25 August: My arms were completely clean and the skin looked beautiful. A number of wart-like growths on my hands and face, which had arisen during the period I had used the hormonal ointment a year earlier, also almost completely disappeared. Swollen moles on my face shrank. A lump on my forefinger joint disappeared. A wart under my arm almost completely disappeared. The old urine also smelled better.

I feel much better since I started using urine therapy. I can imagine that the pharmaceutical industry is not thrilled with this therapy, but that is their problem. Hopefully, people will quickly realize that medication does not have to be expensive, and that we always have it at our side. What has happened to me in four weeks is incredible, and so concretely observable!"

Mr. D.v.K., The Netherlands

"I started using urine therapy when I stopped smoking. I had read that urine therapy has a detoxifying effect, and that was just what I needed. I carefully started drinking the urine in small sips (literally shivering with disgust), massaging myself with five-day-old urine, and even sniffing it into my nostrils. The whole day I thought I smelled urine everywhere – a strange experience! After a few days my kidneys started to hurt, as if somebody were wringing them out by squeezing them. I regularly suffered from shooting pains and after a few days my urine contained fine grit. The grit could have been caused by the contraction of the kidneys, but I cannot be sure of this.

After a week, I had enough of this and so I stopped. After eight weeks I cautiously started again: the first few mornings I only rinsed with urine and thereafter started to gargle. From time to time I drank a small sip; I started to massage my face with fresh urine, and later with old urine.

After two days, I noticed that the urine had an unusual effect on my skin. My pores, which were often oily, were much cleaner and my skin softer.

This second attempt at using urine therapy went much better. After a few days, I started drinking urine. I also drink some of my last urine before going to bed, and this seems to make my morning urine lighter in colour and milder in taste.

After five days I started to have bad breath, and I sometimes had a grey film on my tongue. I had the feeling that my body was being cleansed (apparently through the breathing process). This was inconvenient when I was in the company of other people: I constantly had to use breath fresheners or mouthwash.

After a week, my lymph glands were swollen, especially in my right underarm. For years, I had a small, hard lump under my arm. This had become a soft bump half the size of a hard-boiled egg. It was painful and frightening.

I felt uneasy about the swollen areas under my arms and slept poorly. Two nights later, however, I felt much better. The bump under my right arm was still swollen, but it had decreased in size. On the other hand, I had severe pain under both of my arms, and from time to time in my groin. I started a urine fast.

Two days later, I still had a grey film in my mouth and probably still had bad breath. I took a break from urine therapy: for one day, I did not drink urine or massage with it. Strange – it seemed like I was more tired, as if a kind of clarity disappeared.

The swelling under my arm had almost completely disappeared! I felt a bump the size of a pin-head instead of a large bean. Fantastic!

A day later, the small bump had completely disappeared. I fasted the entire day on urine and a few glasses of water. Another hard bump in my underarm was becoming softer. The hard bump suddenly shrank to one third its size and it was as if I had a marble under my arm.

Ten days later, I started drinking a cup of urine every morning and used it to wash my face and underarms. My skin was still grainy, my pores clearly undergoing a cleansing process. Sometimes when I looked in the mirror, I really noticed how good my skin looked. The rest of the day I also regularly drank my urine, particularly before going to bed. My urine is now almost always light in colour (also in the morning) and smells and tastes milder.

The large lump is practically gone, and the small bump has not even left a trace. I believe that my body has found a balance and has got used to my daily dose of urine."

Ms. J.P., The Netherlands

"I have been using urine therapy for almost a year and have achieved the following successes:

I successfully treated an earache by putting a wad of cotton soaked in urine in my ear. I was able to rid myself of infections by soaking a plaster in old urine and placing this on the infected area. I got rid of neck warts by wiping them off with old urine. The pain from stinging nettle disappeared with the application of fresh urine. Yellow skin and calluses improved. I made it through the entire winter without a stuffed nose or the common cold. If I feel a cold coming on, I sniff urine, the mucus breaks up and after fifteen minutes I'm back to normal. Dry skin is a part of the past. Fasting on urine is easier and more effective. Hair becomes soft. Fever or flu lasts only twenty-four hours. To fight constipation, I drink one-day-old urine.

Furthermore: I rinse off with urine after showering. Once every few months I use henna with old urine for my hair. I give myself enemas with fresh or old urine. Old urine on a wad of cotton helps to cleanse the face. I also take foot baths in old urine (I save the urine in an earthenware pot with a lid).

Urine therapy has helped me get rid of a virus (CMV). Once a week, I am massaged with urine. Afterwards, I sleep soundly."

Mr. J.K., The Netherlands

"I started using urine therapy a month ago, first externally and later internally. The first few days I only drank one sip, and have now increased that to two cups a day. Up until now, I have benefited tremendously.

The eczema on both of my legs and hips was cured within one week. A wart on my forehead and warts on my hands were gone after two weeks. To my amazement and relief, an internal lump on my scrotum has completely disappeared. It was not that difficult for me to start using urine therapy; I just had to get used to the idea."

Mr. H.V., The Netherlands

"Last year, I started washing my hair with urine. I still do, because my limp, soft hair has more body than when I use shampoo.

I have been drinking urine for six months. The first time I drank it, I mixed my urine with water because I thought it was disgusting, but since then I have got used to the taste and even think it tastes good.

I am in good health, but two or three times a year I have the flu and have to stay in bed for a few days. I started drinking my urine particularly during these periods to see if it could help strengthen my resistance to the flu virus. I was greatly disappointed when I felt the flu coming on. I thought, "I was wrong – it doesn't work." However, I rested up for one afternoon and felt fine. This happened again the second time the flu was going around. I stayed in bed for one day, took it easy and felt completely healthy. This never would have happened so quickly in previous years.

Three weeks ago, I accidentally spilled boiling oil onto my hand. I immediately ran ice cold water over my hand. "I need a miracle drug," I thought, "but what?" Of course: urine! Fortunately, I had not urinated in the previous few hours, so that was no problem. I hesitated – shouldn't I let the urine cool down? When I placed my hand in the bucket of urine, it felt healing. I later applied Propolis to the burned area, an ointment which contains Urea Pura and Allantoin (both of which are found in urine). I had second-degree burns. Because I was afraid that the burn would leave a large scar on my hand, I wrapped a bandage soaked in urine around my hand at night and covered this with cling film. I never saw a wound heal so beautifully!"

Ms. I.M., The Netherlands

"A year ago, I was constantly fatigued and sick, had little resistance to illness and was susceptible to every flu that went around. I regularly suffered from stomach cramps, neck and shoulder disorders and forgetfulness.

My general practitioner could not find anything wrong with me. I went to an orthomolecular doctor, who ran a blood test and discovered that I had fungus in my blood, including candida. The fungal infection interfered with my kidney and liver functions, the gall production was too low and there was too much calcium in my blood.

The doctor prescribed an anti-candida diet, nutritional supplements and vitamins. I had heard about urine therapy, and decided to try it instead. I fasted on urine and spring water.

Four days later, I had my blood tested again. My doctor was dumfounded, as the fasting cure so clearly improved the quality of my blood. My immune system started to fight the fungus. New blood photos showed that the calcium was no longer present in my blood and that the intestinal flora had improved.

I continued the cure for three weeks and ate bread without yeast, vegetables and fruit and every morning I drank a glass of urine. I kept getting better, had much more energy and needed less sleep. After these three weeks I switched over to the anti-candida diet plus one glass of morning urine per day. I never felt better!

Besides the practice of drinking urine, what we eat is also very important, certainly in fighting candida disorders."

Ms. M.L., Ireland

"I recently heard about you and the therapy you work with. I want to let you know that in this part of Ireland where I live, till recently baby's were washed with urine. Also, children were often told to use their pee whenever they got wounded or cut in the fields. Unfortunately also here 'modern' life takes its toll and people start to think their old methods are primitive."

Mr. G.K.T., India

"About four years ago I got attracted towards this therapy and was thrilled by its wonderful results. I was suffering from amoebic dysentery since the last 20 years and my physicians had assured me that it will accompany me forever! I was also having eczema since more than 40 years. To my utter surprise I got rid of both major diseases by this wonderful remedy 'Auto Urine Therapy'. You will be further surprised to know that there are some side effects too; but not of the usual harmful nature, which you very often suffer in allopathic treatment. I suffered from falling hair and dandruff. I always used to have cracks in my feet and even on my lips in all the seasons. Likewise I had stomatitis (ulcers in the mouth) once in a few months regularly. I got rid of all the above complaints and ailments unknowingly, as beneficial side effects of this therapy! I have grown younger by many years, and today I am having vigour stamina and energy which I didn't have thirty years before! My wife says, I was not so young, energetic and sexy even in my young days! All these benefits on a wholesale basis were achieved by Auto Urine Therapy of few months."

(From: *Wonders of Uropathy*, G.K. Thakkar, see *Bibliography*)

Mr. J.W., United States

"At the International Conference on Complementary Medicine in Madras, I was sitting next to a physician from Israel who had come to India with an interest in working with lepers. Literature on urine therapy was passed to us which mentioned that urine had been used successfully in the treatment of leprosy. Naturally, he was interested in learning more about it. And of course there is really only one way a person can know about something like urine therapy. We both laughed…

It just so happened that I was coming down with travellers diarrhea. So I thought I would put the unmentionable therapy to the test. I did and I have to admit that first cupful is etched in my memory. Needless to say, I didn't die, I got over my problem very quickly and will never know for sure if it was the urine that did it. After that first shot, the rest was downhill.

I can testify with absolute confidence that the practice of drinking my morning overflow has benefited me greatly not only physically but in mind and spirit. It has made a steady and profound improvement in my health. I am not as moody as I used to be and this has been corroborated by my friends. I've been without any viral conditions since I began, but more importantly I am confident that this practice will help keep me healthy."

(From: *Widening Circle*; A Newsletter from John M. Wynhausen, Doctor of Chiropractic, 1992)

Mr. R.L., The Netherlands

"Since I heard about urine therapy through Armstrong's book, I often used it for oncoming colds, the flu, throataches – and it worked!"

6.3 Immunity-Related Diseases: Cancer, Allergies, AIDS

Urine therapy and cancer

Urine therapy has proven effective in the treatment of many cases of cancer. This does not make urine therapy into a miracle cure for cancer. Cancer is a severe, chronical disease and a lot of commitment, trust and patience are required to achieve any physical healing results. Urine therapy can be very helpful in either alleviating some of the symptoms and reducing pain, and sometimes it actually seems to promote complete healing of the physical manifestation of the disease, the tumor itself.

There are many case-histories of people healed from cancer with the help of urine therapy, to be found throughout the literature on urine therapy. In most of these cases, an intensive form of treatment was followed: fasting on urine and water combined with long massages with old urine.

The reasons for urine therapy being so effective in treating cancer are not yet fully known. Nevertheless, it has become clear through scientific research that there are many substances to be found in urine which have proven anti-cancer properties (see *Chapter 5. A Natural Pharmacy: Medical and Scientific Aspects of Urine Therapy*). Apart from that, urine therapy seems to enhance the strength of the immune system and since cancer is related to a weakening of the body's natural immunity, this immunity enhancing factor could be considered to be quite important. Part of the explanation of urine therapy as such an excellent natural cancer treatment seems to be found in its immense nutritional benefits. Urine contains innumerable easily assimilable nutrients, the ingestion of which helps the body saving its energy it would otherwise spend on metabolic processes needed when eating and drinking normal food and drinks. These nutrients are absorbed both in the intestines and though the skin through the required body massages.

The testimonials given below may serve as an illustration to these remarks on urine therapy and its healing effects on cancer.

Ms. T.A., Australia

"In 1988 I myself had cancer in the bowel, liver and lymph system. For the cancer in the bowel I had three operations within three months, after which I was only skin and bone. For the liver and lymph glands I was offered chemotherapy, which I declined. All the anesthetics, antibiotics and post-operative drugs had

weakened the immune system to rock bottom, and because of this I had already started to lose great bunches of hair.

I had asked God, in prayer, to bring me anything I needed to get well again, and the very next morning I was given by a friend a "Water of Life" book, which in medical terms is uropathy or urine therapy, written by J.W. Armstrong. Such is God's immediate response!

I thanked the Father within me, and I knew that what I had read would totally heal me, if I now applied it to my own situation and condition. I decided not to tell my doctor or anyone until I felt totally healed. I did not want any discouragement or negative influence. I kept up with meditation and relaxation, my usual wheatgrass juice, mixed with lettuce juice to make it more palatable, and other veggie juices. Plenty of salads and greens, no meat, no cooked foods, no dairy products, oils or fats for three months, to heal the liver. Daily rubbings of my whole body, including hair and scalp, with urine. As J.W. Armstrong wrote, and as the Bible says, "Anoint thy body!" The skin is an absorbing organ for the lymph glands. I would do this in the afternoon, and shower the next morning. I also drank my own "Water of Life" in between meals, early morning and during the night, up to seven glasses per day.

Nine months later I went to the doctor, looking and feeling well, which was a great surprise to him. He thought I had already died. A blood test showed no remaining trace of cancer any more."

Mr. J.W., United States

"The seeds of my venture into urine therapy were planted during the Christmas holidays before leaving on my trip to India in early January 1991. I read a very stimulating account by Professor Evangelos D. Danopoulos, M.D. who had successfully treated liver and other cancers using urea and creatine, major components of urine. Professor Danopoulos writes: "The story of my use of urea in the treatment of cancer began in 1954 when I discovered that urine has anti-cancer effect. After long research I discovered that the anti-cancer agent in urine is urea. In 1969, I began to treat cancer patients with oral urea with notable success in primary liver cancer or more often with liver metastases. Also it was soon found that injections of 15% to 50% urea in normal saline into and around skin cancers and malignant breast tumors were most effective." He goes on to relate the further development of using urea and creatine to successfully treat other types of cancer."

(From: *Widening Circle*; A Newsletter from John M. Wynhausen, Doctor of Chiropractic, 1992)

Ms. I.A., Israel

"In 1988 a tumor was discovered on my liver. Since I was already familiar with urine therapy and had often used it, I immediately decided to start drinking my urine. After a period of fasting of almost 4 weeks on predominantly urine and water and occasionally some juices, the whole tumor was gone. In this period I also worked on non-physical levels to support the healing process.

The doctors concluded their diagnosis must have been wrong. Nobody will ever know for sure whether it was just an abscess or cancer, because I had refused to do a biopsy on me. Anyway, I recovered quickly and in the last week of my fast I even often swam a couple of kilometers a day.

I believe that God has separated urine from the feces so we can take the urine in again – fresh, pure and sterile – whenever we need it; as a preventative, but also to remind us that not everything is the way we think it is…."

(From: *The Alchemy of Urine; From Witches' Brew to the Golden Elixir; A Diary*, Immanu-El Adiv, Jerusalem (Israel) 1992, version shortened by author)

Ms. R.Y., Belgium

"I started urine therapy as a result of a breast tumor I had had for a number of years. I drink six glasses of urine daily and rub it into my skin. From time to time I do a fasting cure for two or three days. A couple of times the cure caused me to vomit terribly. I also use urine compresses at night.

The initial results were surprisingly convincing. The tumor reduced in size, the skin in that area regained its colour, the condition of my blood improved and according to a *Touch for Health* measurement, my energy on all levels was strong (it was previously quite weak). My skin and hair have noticeably improved. My eyes have improved and so have my ears, as I inject a few drops of urine into my ears and massage them.

The only thing I miss is the laxative effect of urine, and so I sometimes give myself an enema.

Now, however, I seem to miss noticeable progress,

even though I continue to use urine therapy. For one week, I had a strong aversion to urine and doubted whether it could help me. That has passed, and I now realize that working with urine therapy is not as simple as I initially thought.

I regularly tell others about urine therapy, particularly for external skin problems. People are more willing to try urine externally than internally. Whenever I hear their reactions, I often think: If urine works as well internally as it does externally, then it is a fantastic remedy."

Mr. X., India

"The patient was around 60 years. There were ulcers and fissures on the tongue and in the mouth. In a corner of the mouth, there was a small tumor, which was diagnosed as cancer. Cobalt-ray treatment was given. This was followed by a terrible feeling of burning and soreness inside.

The patient thought of resorting to Water of Life treatment and came to me. I examined all reports and the details of the treatment given. I then prescribed this treatment: To take self-urine into the mouth, rinse the mouth with it and then to spit it out; this, five times a day, every time for 5 to 7 minutes; and then to drink the remaining urine every time. The patient had a little inflammation around the throat and under the ear. Urine was to be rubbed very lightly on these parts every morning and evening. One month's treatment showed a noteworthy improvement, with less

inflammation. The pain and soreness in the mouth had lessened, and in that month the patient maintained status quo in weight, without losing it as he had been doing. The experiment was continued."

(From: *Auto Urine Therapy; Science & Practice*, Vaidya Pragjibhai Mohanji Rathod, Bhavnagar (India) 1988)

Urine therapy and allergies

Nowadays, an immense part of the population seems to suffer from allergies in one form or another. Allergies range from relatively simple forms (such as mild reactions on dust particles) to more complex forms (such as migraine, hay fever certain asthmatic conditions) and extremely complex forms (such as combined food allergies and multiple allergies in syndromes like M.E. (chronic fatigue syndrome). Also many skin disorders are related to allergic reactions (e.g. sun allergy, certain rashes, allergic eczema, neurodermitis, etc.).

Treatments with allopathic chemical medicines have, certainly on the long term, often proven ineffective. They can suppress certain symptoms temporarily, but the symptoms usually come back even stronger or at other locations in the body. Nowadays, because of the increasing complexity of allergy conditions, doctors often cannot even find out any more what their patients are allergic to.

At the same time, urine is scientifically shown to contain a wide range of anti-bodies. These specific anti-allergen antibodies are made by the body itself. When they are re-introduced back into the body, the allergic reaction is stopped. Urine therapy provides several very simple forms of doing this. With urine therapy there is no need to identify the allergy-causing factor.

The practice of injecting urine to treat allergies has in several scientific research projects as well as through many years of practical application proven its tremendous value and effectiveness (see *Chapter 5. A Natural Pharmacy: Medical and Scientific Aspects of Urine Therapy*).

Given below are some testimonials from people with allergy related disorders.

Ms. T.M.K., The Netherlands

"A year ago, I started drinking one glass of morning urine per day on an empty stomach. I still do, not because it tastes good but because this has caused a number of symptoms from which I was suffering to diminish and even disappear.

The first few sips were nothing like broth, like everybody says. It simply tasted disgusting – salty, bitter and lukewarm. I followed a healthy diet, so that was not the cause. Even so, it was not too disgusting to drink, and I was sufficiently motivated.

I have had M.E. (chronic fatigue syndrome) for a good four years. Besides being chronically fatigued, I often contract infections (particularly of the bronchial tubes), suffer from muscle and joint pain, and have splitting headaches which last for up to five days. The past few years, I was sick every six weeks for three consecutive weeks – a nasty cold complete with infected canker sores, followed by bronchitis.

This year, since I started drinking urine, I have had the flu a few times, but without that horrible stuffed nose and bronchitis, and only had one infected canker sore. The muscle and joint pain gradually diminished and is now completely gone! My headaches have not

disappeared, but they do not last as long, are less severe and occur less often. The fatigue has not decreased, but I do sleep better.

I must add that none of this can be proven scientifically. Maybe these healing processes spontaneously and magically occurred – who knows?

I clearly remember that the first few weeks after I started drinking my morning urine, I had an unusual vibrating feeling in my head, as if a current of energy had been released. It was a very relaxing feeling. This lasted a few months, and I later heard that other 'urine-drinkers' experience this as well. The most amazing thing is that the head colds have completely disappeared. My intuition tells me that urine therapy definitely helped cure me of those nasty head colds.

I believe that my body lets me know when I have drunk the exact amount of urine that I need. I always get the feeling, "Hold it, stop! Enough is enough." If I keep drinking to see how my body will react, I usually start to gag.

I practice urine therapy as a kind of ritual, with a fixed order of doing things. For example, I could never leave the lavatory with my glass of urine and drink it in the living room or wait until it has cooled down – I would not be able to drink it. I stay seated on the toilet and drink my urine lukewarm until I reach the 'enough is enough' point. I sometimes drink a few sips of water afterwards. Drinking a glass of spring water or weak herbal tea in the evening makes the urine taste milder.

To your health!"

Ms. B.A., England

"I had been suffering from migraine for twenty years. Because I also suffered from rheumatoid arthritis, I was often taking painkillers. Then I started drinking my urine. A few months later, my arthritis had disappeared and so did my headaches."

Ms. E.C., The Netherlands

"For a long time I have been suffering from strong hay fever attacks. Among the symptoms are itching and swollen eyes, asthmatic conditions and constant sneezing.

I started to clean my eyes every morning with some cotton wool soaked in urine. From that moment on, the itching and swelling of the eyes disappeared, the sneezing stopped and the asthma attacks have become bearable."

Mr. L.C., Germany

"I was regularly suffering from sun allergy. Since I heard about urine therapy, I just rub my urine on the affected skin parts and usually the allergy rapidly disappears and the skin stops itching."

Mr. X., India

"The patient, whom I am going to talk about, was about 40 years old. He had been getting attacks for the preceding 10 years. The attack began with a dripping nose and sneezing and was then followed by breathlessness. This had been diagnosed as some kind of allergy. Whenever there was an attack, the doctor would give the patient an injection of adrenalin, and the patient would feel relief. This cycle was often repeated.

I decided to give him Water of Life treatment. The patient agreed to abide by the restrictions in diet which I suggested him. I prescribed two things: 1) To drink his urine twice daily in doses of 10 oz, once on an empty stomach and next at night, before going to bed, and 2) To heat fresh urine and massage the chest, the back, the neck, etc. with it. I also prescribed rapeseed oil to be taken internally.

Considerable relief was felt at the end of a month's treatment."

(From: *Auto Urine Therapy; Science & Practice*, Vaidya Pragjibhai Mohanji Rathod, Bhavnagar (India) 1988)

Urine therapy and AIDS

A number of personal experiences from people with HIV follow below. I have already mentioned that a urine therapy support group exists in New York City with some 700 members. (Also in Los Angeles recently such a support group has been started.) This group has become so large partly due to the inspiration from Quique Palladino, a man who believed that his remarkable remission of AIDS symptoms was caused by his use of urine. He has conducted a great deal of research on the scientific foundation of urine therapy and in doing so found and made available extremely useful information. Although his enthusiasm was great and the improvements remarkable, Quique died four years ago from AIDS. His story would not be complete without these data. Following the urgent advice of a doctor, Quique decided to take medication for a short period of time in order to fight an acute infection. Because he knew that drinking urine and taking allopathic medication do not mix, he temporarily stopped urine therapy. Due to further complications, Quique decided to use AZT. He died a few months later.

Urine therapy did not cause Quique Palladino to go into permanent remission. His story demonstrates, however, that the use of urine therapy can bring about considerable alleviation of certain symptoms, and therefore an improvement in the quality of life. The other short reports from people with AIDS who believe they were helped by urine therapy are only an indication of the possible positive effects of urine therapy in the fight against AIDS-specific symptoms. The case histories given below are by no means meant to suggest that urine therapy provides a cure for AIDS! Further research and good documentation as to where and to which extent these beneficial effects of urine therapy can be relied upon, are desired and necessary.

Mr. Quique Palladino, United States

"She didn't like me at all – laughing and snickering at her and her partner, as I sat there on the hardwood floor. After all, who would take anyone seriously talking about drinking one's urine to cure any disease…!

My main concern at the time was how was I going to handle this diagnosis of full-blown AIDS and with what level of "spirituality" was I going to handle an oral, palatal, Kaposi's Sarcoma lesion that was supposed to spread relentlessly throughout my body. I was told just two months prior that the prognosis could be about two years, more if fortunate, and to seriously consider preparing a "living will"…

For obvious reasons, I seemed to be much more tolerant to the idea of applying urine topically for all sorts of conditions. Eczema, boils, burns, cuts, infections, and lesions to poison ivy, hives and fungal infections are just a few that are alleviated or eradicated. I was always a strong advocate of herbal remedies and other gentle and natural forms of dealing with diseased conditions of the body, so douching for yeast infections, taking enemas, gargling, and soaking an appendage, all with one's own urine, seemed to awaken some ancient, primordial, almost hidden secret from deep inside me. Then I remembered my father's account of an Italian immigrant who drank a cup of his urine every day at break time in the factory, swearing it was the safest and most effective way to heal a large stomach ulcer.

Then an article in *Time* (October 24, 1977) came to mind about how India's ex-Prime Minister, Morarji Desai, startled a meeting of India's Tuberculosis Association by informing his audience that "self-urine" therapy was a cure for cancer and cataracts and that he had cured his own brother of tuberculosis that way. Yes, and he has been drinking a glass-full of his own urine for the "past five or six years."

My right foot was the epitome of necrosis. For months the doctors had prescribed many different medicated creams for a voracious case of athletes feet/ringworm. Nothing seemed to work; after all, the root of the problem is the immune system not functioning at full capacity. When Margie spoke about how wonderfully she had cleared up a terrible vaginal yeast infection in just three days by simply douching with her own urine in a solution of Golden Seal, the wheels started turning. I couldn't wait to go home to put my urine on the foot. That evening was the first time in many months that that tingling itch did not drive me into a frenzy! I actually got a full night of sleep! Stopping the applications only yielded regression of the foot condition, so I willingly sprayed the foot every morning…

Not only did the ringworm condition totally disappear after a few weeks, but the dry, cracked and painful skin all around my toes and bottom of the foot had totally changed in colour and texture! New skin had grown in and was soft as a baby's. It had a beautiful new flushed, almost orange-like colour and just did not appear to be my own skin! I was convinced that there was something to this liquid we all produce in our bodies and would have been very foolish not to pursue it any further.

I anxiously began to research the field of the use of autogenous fluids and shortly thereafter, decided that recycling my own urine was really a harmless form of auto-toleration based on theories not much different than those in the science of homoeopathy.

I then graduated to drinking up to 8 ounces of my urine daily. I learned that the morning urine is the most potent (in beneficial effects as well as in consistency), for during the night when the body is totally relaxed, more healing and hormonal processes take place. Over the next 7 months, the Kaposi's Sarcoma lesion became increasingly smaller until it has disappeared totally! The mouth ulcers that used to plague me, stinging during meals, have not returned even once. I used to have monthly outbreaks of genital herpes, but I am

elated to say that autogenous uropathy has produced a state of tolerance even against the herpes virus that sooner or later, in conjunction with Epstein-Barr (EBV), Cytomegalovirus (CMV), and Papilloma Virus would have surely complicated my existence and further weakened my immune system… just a matter of time. I have *never* felt better in my life and I no longer fear for my life.

For those with any AIDS-related sensitivities or concerns, auto-urine treatment, whether by injection or by drinking, seems to enhance or stimulate the immune system, mostly of the T-cell population. Being HIV antibody positive is not necessarily an evil; rather, it is a sign that the body is fighting and reacting to the antigen. Recycling those specific antibodies in your urine can increase the body's ability to use those antibodies, helping to return the body to the healthy balance *on its own*, achieving restored cell-mediated immunity. I am convinced that antibiotics, vaccines, serums, boosters, and inoculations of many types only exacerbate any imbalances and complicate the ability of the body to fight its own battles.

Being a PWA (Person with AIDS) should have brought me many infections, major and minor, but after a year and a half I have not even had the flu or a common cold. My energy level, although it was never really depressed, has actually increased and my body requires much less sleep than over the previous 7 years of my life.

I strongly believe in the holistic adage that "What cannot be cured by the forces of the body, cannot be cured by the forces outside the body." What relationship can be more streamlined, more intimate, more holographic than the actual vibrations of your own body fluids!"

(From: "Urine-Therapy, Drinking from Thine Own Cistern", Quique Palladino, PWA Coalition Newsline, Nr. 37, October 1988, p.41-44, version shortened by author)

Ms. R.G., The Netherlands

"More than two years ago, a friend told me about urine therapy. I immediately started a fast for a few days and afterwards felt much better. Moreover, I had gained a great deal of faith from this experience: I suddenly realized what a great influence attitude has on health and well-being.

Although I knew I was HIV-positive, I did not think about the possible consequences. At one point, I started suffering from itching around my vagina; my doctor told me that this symptom often occurred in people who were HIV-positive. The doctor gave me an ointment, but I soon stopped using it, as I could not stand the idea of being dependent on an ointment. I realized that since urine flows in and around that area anyway, perhaps it could help take away the itching. Apparently, the thought alone was sufficient – the symptom quickly disappeared.

Some time later, I started suffering from sinusitis again, an old and familiar ailment. At that time, I did not drink my urine every day. Over a period of a few weeks, the sinusitis developed into a nasty, chronic, common cold. I could not shake this cold, and constantly had a splitting headache. My homeopathic remedies were ineffective, and so I stopped taking them and at the same time started drinking my urine. At that time my urine was quite dark. A friend told me this indicated a loss of vitamin B, and so I started taking extra vitamin B and C. This was the only 'extra' remedy that I took. I dripped old urine into my nose and supplemented the treatment with meditation and breathing exercises, such as pranayama. I gradually got better, and after a while all of the symptoms disappeared.

This was a rough period for me. I was confronted with my fears, especially my fear of death. Afterwards, however, I was not afraid any more. I was very peaceful, had more faith, and developed a new attitude towards life, all of which I nurtured with meditation. I learned to let go of my expectations, even of meditation. Of course, at times my faith also failed me.

Six months later I developed a number of spots under my arms. It seemed to be a kind of allergy, and it itched like crazy. I scratched many scabs open and it was very painful. When I started to dab the spots with urine, the scabs closed up in no time and the spots disappeared. Since then, I use urine for every scrape and wound, and it works excellently. I massage urine into my face, and blemishes disappear quickly. Whenever friends ask me how come I look so good, I just answer, "Urine does it!"

I also plan to get my T-cell count tested regularly to see if anything has changed.

I trust urine therapy based on what I have heard and read, but most of all based on my own experiences. I realize that only my own experiences can teach me anything, not within a month or a year, but possibly over a longer period of time."

Mr. E.J.P., The Netherlands

"I think we can also expect a lot from this method in the fight against AIDS. I have seen AIDS patients start urine therapy in spite of such trying circumstances, and these experiences are certainly encouraging. Two years ago, a friend of mine was examined for a stomach ulcer and was diagnosed as having 'full blown' AIDS (she had a T4 of 80; according to her doctors, she had three to six months to live). She reacted badly to AZT and could not tolerate other medication. Two to four months after starting urine therapy, the spots on her skin disappeared, including the candida fungus which had turned her throat entirely white. Her energy returned, probably due to urine therapy combined with a healthy combination of plant-based remedies which strengthened her resistance. Now, more than two years later, she is entirely capable of maintaining her household and caring for her child. These last two years have certainly not been easy, partly due to the fact that the doctors did not cooperate. They kept warning her that without AZT, and considering her general condition, she would not live longer than six months."

Mr. B., United States

"I am a PWA (person with AIDS) and I have been doing urine therapy for three months. My fatigue and dizziness dissipated within the first month. I experienced intense eye itchiness. A few drops of fresh urine stopped it immediately. If I forget to take the urine one day, the next day I will pay for it with fatigue. Also my lymph gland swelling is reduced by 50%."

(From: *Urine-Therapy: It May Save Your Life*, Dr. Beatrice Bartnett, Margate Fla. 1989, p.22)

Mr. L., United States

"I have been doing urine therapy for four months now. I am a PWA. My only symptom was a low T-cell count. My last test showed my T-cell count went up from 285 to 489."

(From: *Urine-Therapy: It May Save Your Life*, Dr. Beatrice Bartnett, Margate Fla. 1989, p.22)

Mr. D., United States

"I am a PWA. Three months prior to starting urine therapy I experienced heavy night sweats, and I needed 18 hours of sleep daily! Also my skin was very dry and ashy looking. All these symptoms got resolved within 10 days of urine therapy. I now play one hour of basketball every day. What a difference!"

(From: *Urine-Therapy: It May Save Your Life*, Dr. Beatrice Bartnett, Margate Fla. 1989, p.23)

Mr. M., United States

"I am a PWA and my major problem was parasites. My stool sample contained pus, large amounts of yeast and several parasites. My last test came back totally clear. No more pus and no more parasites!"

(From: *Urine-Therapy: It May Save Your Life*, Dr. Beatrice Bartnett, Margate Fla. 1989, p.23)

Mr. S., United States

"I am a PWA and have been doing urine therapy for two and one-half months. My Lymphadenopathy was gone within 48 hours after starting the urine. I had a severe acne problem on my back. After five weeks the skin is clear. My energy level increased enormously within a few days of drinking my urine."

(From: *Urine-Therapy: It May Save Your Life*,
Dr. Beatrice Bartnett, Margate Fla. 1989, p.24)

A case history from the Swiss Dr.med. U.E. Hasler:

"Mr.S: The patient was HIV-positive and was suffering from several AIDS-related symptoms, such as oral and anal fungus infections, tiredness, red and itching eyes, difficulties to get moving. Subjectively the patient felt healthy again after practicing urine therapy for several months, there was no longer any evidence of the presence of the AIDS-virus in his blood. Without any problems the patient returned to a heavy work schedule, he had the same amount of energy and vitality as he used to have to do his work.

(Also this case I mention with the greatest caution; nevertheless I heard about similar positive experiences with urine therapy in the USA.)"

(From: *Die Apotheke in uns*, Dr.med. U.E. Hasler,
Heidelberg 1994)

7. THE WATER OF AUSPICIOUSNESS: Shivambu Kalpa Vidhi

7.1   Introduction to the Indian Text

Professor Athavale, an Indian Cultural History and Sanskrit scholar, discovered the text *Shivambu Kalpa Vidhi*, an ancient document which discusses urine therapy. This is a manuscript from the extensive collection of His Holiness Shankaracharya of Dwarka.

As discussed in Chapter 3, this document was written for those who studied yoga and meditated, within the Eastern philosophy and ideology. The imagery used in this document is aimed at these people, and may seem exaggerated to the modern Western reader. However, this religious aspect aside, the text is full of valuable and practical information and is of great interest.

For the following translation I used the three already existing translations from R.V. Karlekar, Arthur Lincoln Pauls and from the book *Auto-Urine Therapy* (see bibliography). I relied on Arthur Lincoln Pauls' commentary in his book *Shivambu Kalpa* for some lucid explanations of certain parts of this document.

This ancient text suggests using old, boiled down urine for massage. The text states that the external use of urine which has not been boiled down can even have harmful consequences. However, research and experience have demonstrated that this is not the case and that fresh urine as well as urine which is not boiled down, but which is at least four days old, produces excellent results during external use. This is also true for boiled down urine, as suggested in this text.

7.2   The Entire Document on Urine Therapy from the Damar Tantra

Shivambu Kalpa Vidhi
Verses 1 – 4
Oh Parvati! (The God Shiva speaks to his wife Parvati.) Those who practice this method can enjoy the fruits of their meditation and this method. For this, certain actions have been recommended along with certain types of utensils. The Shivambu is to be drunk from pots made of gold, silver, copper, brass, iron, tin, glass, earth, bamboo, bones, leather, or a bowl made of plantain leaves.

The urine should be collected in any one of the above mentioned utensils and should be drunk. However, earthen pots are the best for use.

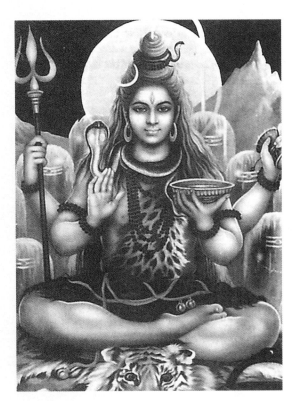

Shiva, one of the most important gods from the Indian pantheon. In India, urine is often called Shivambu *by urine therapists, which means as much as 'the water of Shiva' or 'the water of auspiciousness'.*

Verse 5

The follower of the therapy should avoid pungent, salty ingredients in his meals. He should not over-exert himself. He should follow a balanced and light diet. He should sleep on the ground, and control the senses.

Verse 6

Such a trained man gets up in the early morning when three quarters of the night has passed, stands facing the east and passes urine.

Verse 7

The first and concluding flow of the urine is to be left out, and the intermediate flow of urine is to be collected. This is the best method.

Verse 8

The follower of the therapy should only use his own urine; it is called Shivambudhara. However, just as the mouth and the tail of the serpent contain poison, similarly the first and the concluding flow of urine are not wholesome.

Verse 9

Shivambu is a divine nectar! It is capable of abolishing old age and various types of diseases and ailments. The follower should first ingest his urine and then start his meditation.

Verse 10

After getting out of bed, the face and the mouth should be washed with water. Afterwards, one should drink one's own urine quite willingly and cheerfully.

All the ailments subject to from the very birth will be completely cured.

Verse 11

If this method is followed for one month, one's body will be internally cleansed. Drinking it for two months stimulates and energizes the senses.

Verse 12

If this method is followed for three months, all types of ailments will disappear and all miseries will evaporate. After following this method for five months, the follower will be completely healthy and will be bestowed with divine eyesight.

Verse 13

After six months of following this therapy, the follower will be exceptionally intelligent. After seven months, the follower will be extraordinarily strong.

Verse 14

After eight months the human body will possess divine luster like that of shining gold which will be permanent. After nine months of continual use, tuberculosis and leprosy will perish.

Verse 15

After ten months of continual use, the follower becomes practically the treasury of luster and brightness. After eleven months, the follower becomes pure, both externally and internally.

Verse 16

After one year of continual use, the follower acquires solar shining. After two years, the follower can conquer the element of earth.

Verse 17

After three years of practicing this therapy, the follower can conquer the element of water. After four years, the follower can certainly conquer the element of luster.

Verse 18

After five years, the follower can conquer the element of air. Seven years of use makes the follower capable of conquering his ego.

Verse 19

After eight years of working with this method, the follower can conquer all the five important elements of the universe.

Nine years of this method will make the follower immortal.

Verse 20

After ten years of experimentation, it will be possible to float in the air with ease. After eleven years, the follower will be able to listen to the movements of the internal organs of the body.

Verse 21

Experiments for the duration of twelve years will enable one to be as long lived as the moon and the planets. Dangerous animals such as serpents will not effect one in any way; serpents' poison will not kill the follower. One can float on water just as wood floats and he will never drown.

Verses 22, 23

Oh Goddess! I shall tell you of some other aspects of the therapy. Listen to me carefully. If taken for six months continually, the powder of Amrita (Tinospora Condifalia) dissolved in Shivambu will make a man free from human ailments and he will become perfectly happy.

Verse 24

The powder of Haritaki (Terminalia Chebula) mixed with Shivambu should be taken regularly for one year. It puts a stop to old age and disease and if used for one year makes a man exceptionally strong and healthy.

Verse 25

Shivambu should be taken with one gram of sulphur. If this is followed for three years, man may acquire longevity as long as the moon and planets exist. The urine and excreta of such a man may become white and gold.

Verse 26

The stomach powder, Kostha Churna, should be taken with Shivambu continually for a period of twelve years. The tokens of old age such as wrinkles on the skin, grey hair, etc., vanish. Man will have the strength of ten thousand elephants and will live as long as the moon and the planets exist.

Verse 27

The mixture of pepper, terminalia belavica, terminalia chebula, if taken with Shivambu will enable man to acquire divine luster and brightness.

Verses 28, 29

The extract of mica and sulphur should be dissolved in Shivambu and taken regularly. It relieves the ailment of dropsy and rheumatism. Man becomes strong and divinely lustrous. He can enjoy longevity and can compete with death.

Verse 30

A follower who takes Shivambu regularly and avoids pungent, salty and sour things, can promptly enjoy the fruits of his meditation and this method.

Verse 31

He becomes free from human ailments. He assumes divinely lustrous physique like that of Shiva; he can recreate the universe and can lead divinely pleasant life.

Verse 32

A meditator who lives on the juice of neem leaves and Shivambu attains the status of yogi and possesses the divinely pleasant luster full of bliss.

Verse 33

The powder of neem bark and pumpkin gourd dissolved in Shivambu taken for a year relieves man from all types of ailments.

Verse 34

The mixture of lotus roots, mustard seeds and honey should be taken with Shivambu. It makes the human body exceptionally light and energetic.

Verse 35

The fruits of the moha tree and a tri-mixture of the herbs in verse 27, should be taken in equal proportion and dissolved in Shivambu. This is capable of relieving old age and all kinds of diseases.

Verse 36

Rock salt and honey in equal proportions should be taken first in the early morning, followed by Shivambu. This makes man lustrous and he acquires a body with divine attributes.

Verse 37

Sulphur, dried fruit of Amla (Phylonthus Emblica) and nutmeg powder should be mixed together and taken daily, followed by Shivambu. All pains and miseries vanish.

Verse 38

The follower should regularly drink milk and Shivambu. If this is done for seven years, all human ailments perish and the body becomes well nourished and strong.

Verse 39

He who takes Amritaka powder (the extract of tinospora condifolia) and then Shivambu can conquer death.

Verse 40

He who drinks the mixture of Shivambu and honey or sugar is relieved of any type of ailment within a period of six months. His brain power becomes brilliant and his voice becomes melodious.

Verse 41

The powder of dry ginger taken first directly followed by Shivambu definitively relieves any disease.

Verse 42

He who first chews on the leaves of Viter Nirgundi and then drinks Shivambu will be bestowed with divine eyesight.

Verse 43

The powder of mansheel should be dissolved in Shivambu and the solution applied to the body. This makes man free of ailments and his hair becomes black (again).

Verse 44

Now, oh Parvati, I shall tell you about the process of massage.

If such a massage is carried out, the follower can enjoy the fruits of his meditation and his lifestyle and will experience spiritual growth.

Verse 45

The Shivambu should be boiled in an earthen pot and extracted to one fourth its quantity. It should then be allowed to cool. This extract can be used for the body massage.

Verse 46

The following mantra should be recited during the use of Shivambu. When collecting urine in an earthen pot, the following mantra should be recited:

"Om Rhim Klim Bhairavaya Namaha" (salutes to Bhairav).

The pot filled with Shivambu should then be taken into the hands. When drinking urine from the pot the mantra to be recited is

"Om Shrim Klim Uddamaneshwaraya Namah"
(salutes to Uddamaneshwara).

The follower will be away from all sins and defects.

Verse 47

While passing urine, the mantra to be recited is
"Om Sarvam Sristhi Prabhave Rudraya Namaha".
(Salutes to God Rudra).

Verse 48

Shivambu should be applied to the whole body. It is exceptionally nourishing, and can relieve all ailments.

Verse 49

The follower can acquire divine power with this process. A yogi can become the King of Gods. His movements will be unprevented. He will have the strength of ten thousand elephants. He can eat and digest anything.

Verse 50

Urine which has not been boiled down to one fourth its volume should never be applied to the body; if done so, it makes the body weak and invites ailments.

Verse 51

Unboiled urine should never be used for body massage. If the extract of Shivambu is used for the massage, it is very wholesome for the body. The follower can accomplish many things.

Verse 52

The follower can conquer death by drinking Shivambu and massaging with one fourth extract of the same.

Verse 53

His urine and excrement can impart a white colour to gold. If Shiro-Amrit and dew are mixed in the extract of Shivambu and if the mixture is applied to the body, the man will become exceptionally strong and will be free from any type of ailment.

Verse 54

A follower should drink Shivambu every morning regularly for a period of three years. This and avoiding bitter, salty and pungent things in his meals, will enable him to conquer passion.

Verse 55 and 56

Chickpeas should be roasted and taken with unrefined sugar followed by the intake of Shivambu. Urine extract should also be applied to the body. After six months the human body becomes quite light and energetic.

Verse 57

Oh wife of the highest of Gods! Roots of Piper Longum and one gram of black pepper should be taken first and afterwards Shivambu should be drunk. Within one month, the voice will become melodious and all ailments will vanish.

Verse 58

The follower should first take the powder of dry ginger and then drink Shivambu. It makes him exceptionally strong. He may acquire the strength of ten thousand elephants. His youth will even attract divine females.

Verse 59

Oh wife of Shiva! Terminalia Chebula should be roasted and then powdered. It should be taken first, followed by the intake of Shivambu. The follower's body will be cleansed, his mind will be ever cheerful and he can attain divine luster.

Verse 60

He who drinks Shivambu after taking a mixture of equal proportions (powdered) of Amrita, Triphala, Kadu, dried ginger, cumin seeds and the roots of Piper Longum while following a diet of rice and milk will have insight in the Scriptures within one year.

Verse 61

If this experiment is followed for a period of one year, the follower will become very strong and brave. If he follows this for a period of three years, he will become, as it were, a god on earth. He will enjoy the fruits of this practice, will become a good orator and all the universe will be visible to his eyesight.

Verse 62

The follower who drinks the mixture of Shivambu and the powder of the five parts of the Sharapunkha (Devnal) plant will become the master and authority of meditation. He will enjoy utmost pleasure in life.

Verses 63, 64

Oh great Goddess! Shivambu should be taken with the powder of dried ginger, sugar, ghee, honey and the juice of Nirgundi leaves. Within one month, the body becomes healthy and strong and after one year he will enjoy the fruits of this method and meditation.

Verse 65

The follower should take white and black sesame seeds (in equal proportion) mixed with Karanja seeds (Pongamia Glabvi) and the juice of neem leaves. This should be followed by Shivambu, which will enable the follower to achieve the fruits of this method and meditation.

Verses 66, 67

Opium should be roasted on an open fire; 1/32 of this should be taken along with the Shivambu. He will then be able to control ejaculation and will be unconquerable in sexual intercourse. He can control his breath, passion, anger and other mental emotions. He can enjoy longevity.

Verse 68

Oh Goddess! Triphala Churna, Nirgundi leaves and Turmeric should be mixed together, followed by Shivambu. Within a period of three months, the follower of the therapy becomes a symbol of learning and enjoys excellent eyesight. His body becomes divinely lustrous.

Verse 69

Bhringaraj and honey should be mixed and taken first, followed by Shivambu. The follower, after six months, will be free of old age and will have excellent (fore)sight.

Verse 70

The neem bark, roots of Chitraka (Plumago Zeylancia) and the roots of Piper Longum mixed together should be taken with Shivambu and within six months the follower of the therapy attains divine power.

Verse 71

The root of Apamarg (Achyranthus Aspara) and Chakramarda (Chenopadium Album) and the juice of neem leaves should be taken, followed by Shivambu.

Verse 72

He will be relieved from all ailments and the tokens of old age, such as wrinkles and greying hair. He will possess excellent and long eyesight within a distance of miles and miles.

Verse 73

He will be able to listen for a very long distance. He can read the mind of others. O Goddess, even the most beautiful Princess will be attracted to him.

Verse 74

A very small quantity (one grain) of Nerium Odorum should be taken with Shivambu and within a year epilepsy and other mental disorders will disappear.

Verse 75

The juice of white Gunja (Abrus Precatorius), the leaves of Sharapunkha (Devala), seeds of Chenopadium Album and roots of Mahalung should be taken in equal proportions and all mixed into a fine powder.

Verses 76, 77

This powder should be dissolved in Shivambu and small pills be prepared with the mixture. Every day one pill should be taken followed by a sufficient quantity of Shivambu. The follower of this therapy will be relieved from human ailments of all types within one month.

Verse 78

The gum of the Banian tree (Ficus Bengalensis) should be mixed with the powder of the seeds of Karanja (Pongamia Glabra). A small quantity of opium should be added to this mixture. It should be taken early in the morning, followed by Shivambu.

Verse 79

Within six months, the follower of this therapy will become as young as a lad of sixteen years. He can disguise himself by appearance and non-appearance to his desire.

Verse 80

The juice of the leaves of Kavali, honey, sugar and ghee should be mixed together. If it is taken regularly in the morning, the signs of old age disappear promptly.

Verse 81

Cumin seeds, turmeric and white mustard seed should be powdered together and taken regularly. This also helps to conquer old age.

Verse 82

Black Moringa Pterygasperma, Jatamavasi, mustard seeds should be dissolved in honey and ghee and then taken regularly. It gives divine countenance.

Verse 83

Kalnemi Veesh (Guggul) and the roots of Bhargika (Clerodendron Serrotum) should be dissolved in butter, and taken with Shivambu. It will definitely give shining countenance.

Verse 84

Jalakesar moss and the seeds of Sapindus Laurifolius should be dissolved in Shivambu and taken regularly. Within one year old age will be under control and the follower will acquire a radiating personality, like that of the famous King Udayan, the King of the Vatsas.

Verse 85

Oh Goddess, if in the early morning the follower nasalizes his own urine, the ailments arising out of Kapha, Pitta and Vata will vanish. He will have a healthy appetite and his body will become strong and healthy.

Verse 86

If the follower of the therapy massages his body thrice a day and thrice a night with Shivambu, he will definitely enjoy longevity.

Verse 87

Oh Parvati! If he massages his body thrice a day and night with Shivambu, his countenance will be shining and his heart will be strong. His body and muscles will be strong. He will float in pleasure.

Verse 88

Oh Parvati! He who massages his body at least once a day with Shivambu will be full of strength and bravery.

Verse 89

Within three years his body will be shining with luster. He will be well versed in arts and science. He will have an impressive voice with good oratory powers, and will live as long as the moon and planets exist.

Verse 90

Oh Goddess, now I shall narrate the procedure of seasonable behavior with the view to avoiding diseases and ailments.

Verse 91

Oh Parvati, during the Spring the powder of Terminalia Chebula should be taken with honey; dry ginger and honey should also be taken and afterwards Shivambu.

Verse 92

Twenty types of ailments arising from Kapha, twenty-four types of ailments arising from Pitta and eighty types of ailments arising from Vata will vanish with this treatment.

Verse 93

Oh Great Goddess, during the Spring, pungent and spicy foods are to be avoided. This helps to attain sound health.

Verses 94, 95

Oh Great Goddess, during the summer the Haritaki (Terminalia Chebula) and pepper should be taken in equal quantities and should be taken with unrefined sugar followed by Shivambu. This will relieve all kinds of ailments; the body will become light, eyesight will be sharp and at the end the follower will derive the fruits of this method.

Verses 96, 97

During the rainy season (July-August), Haritaki (Terminalia Chebula), rock salt and roots of pepper should be taken in a powder form, followed by the intake of Shivambu. The body will be strong and will attain shining luster. If he takes the powder mixture in milk, even fire will not harm him. He will not be burnt by fire.

Verses 98, 99

During the Sharad season (September-October), Haritaki (Terminalia Chebula), crystal sugar and Terminalia Belavica powder should be mixed together and taken, followed by Shivambu. This method cleanses the body, keeps it free of disease and allows the follower to move quickly. And oh, wife of the King of the Gods, the follower will quickly master the practice of yoga.

Verses 100, 101

During the Hemanta season (November-December), dry ginger, dried fruit of Anvla (Phylonthus Emblica) and Haritaki (Terminalia Chebula) should be mixed into a fine powder followed by Shivambu. If taken regularly, deficiency of minerals in the body is corrected, eyesight brightens, oratory powers and knowledge are acquired.

Verses 102, 103

During the Shishir season (January-February), pepper, Haritaki (Terminalia Chebula) and dry ginger should be mixed and taken, followed by Shivambu. It will cure various diseases, the follower will acquire the strength of a hundred elephants and the signs of old age will vanish. He will attract all living beings.

Verses 104, 105, 106

Oh Goddess, during the process of the intake of Shivambu, the following things should be strictly avoided: vegetables in the form of leaves, flowers or legumes; grains that cause flatulency; and starchy, pungent, sour and salty foods. Sexual intercourse should also be avoided. This will help to accomplish the fruits of this method. Behaving against these rules will put man in unexpected difficulties.

Verse 107

Oh my beloved Parvati! I have narrated the details of Shivambu Kalpa. This is its technique. Attempts should be made to keep it a secret. Do not tell anyone.

Here ends the Chapter on Shivambu Kalpa Vidhi as described in the Damar Tantra.

Bibliography

(based on chronological order of publication)

Urine as An Autotherapeutic Remedy, Dr. Charles H. Duncan, 1918

Die Eigenharnbehandlung, Dr. med. Kurt Herz, 1st edition 1930, 5th edition Karl F. Haug Verlag, Ulm, Heidelberg (Germany) 1980

Der menschliche Harn als Heilmittel; Geschichte. Grundlagen. Entwicklung, Praxis, Martin Krebs, Hippokrates Verlag Marquardt & Cie., Stuttgart (Germany) 1942

The Water of Life, John W. Armstrong, 1st edition England 1944, Health Science Press, Saffron Walden (England) 1990

Manav Mootra, Dr. R.M. Patel, 1st edition 1963, 5th edition Lokseva Kendra Publ., Ahmedabad (India) 1991

Auto-Urine Cure, R.V. Karlekar, Shree Gajanan Book Depot Prakashan, Bombay (India) 1969

Miracles of Urine Therapy, Dr. C.P. Mithal, Pankaj Publications, New Delhi (India) 1978

Shivambu Kalpa, Dr. Arthur L. Pauls, Ortho-Bionomy Publishing, (England) 1978

Amaroli, Dr. Swami Shankardevan Saraswati, Bihar school of yoga, Bihar (India) 1978

Auto-Urine Therapy, Acharya Jagdish B., Jagdish B. Publications, Bombay (India) 1978

The Eating Gorilla Comes in Peace, Bubba Free John, Dawn Horse Press, San Rafael (California, USA) 1979, pp.220-224

"Auto-urotherapy", John R. Herman, New York State Journal of Medicine, vol. 80n no.7 June 1980, pp.1149-1154

Urine Therapy; Self Healing through Intrinsic Medicine, Dr. John F. O'Quinn, Life Science Institute, Fort Pierce (Florida, USA) 1982

Health in Your Hands, Devendra Vora, Gala Publishers, Bombay (India) 1982, pp.3, 122-123

Cancer Cures in Twelve Ways, A.A. Cordero, Science of Nature Healing Center Asia, (Philippines) 1983, pp..395-404

Tibetan Buddhist Medicine and Psychiatry, The Diamond Healing, Terry Clifford, Samuel Weiser Inc. York Beach (USA) 1984

The Miracles of Urine Therapy, Dr. Beatrice Bartnett & Margie Adelman, Water of Life Institute, Hollywood (Florida, USA) 1987

Auto Urine Therapy; Science & Practice, Vaidya Pragjibhai Mohanji Rathod, Swasthvrutta Prakashan, Bhavnagar (India) 1988

"Urine-Therapy, Drinking from Thine Own Cistern", Quique Palladino, PWA Coalition Newsline, Nr. 37, October 1988, pp.41-44 (USA) 1988

Amaroli, Dr. Soleil & Dr. C. T. Schaller, 1st edition 1989, Editions Vivez Soliel, Genève (Switzerland) 1993

Urine-Therapy; It May Save Your Life , Dr. Beatrice Bartnett, Water of Life Institute, Hollywood (Florida, USA) 1989

Auto-Urine Therapy, 'An experienced physician' (anonymous), Gala Publishers, Ahmedabad (India) 1990

P..., Buvez, Guérissez, Claude Gauthier, Editions ABC, Saint-Serrasy (France) 1991

Die Eigenharnbehandlung: nach Dr. med. Kurt Herz; Erfahrungen und Beobachtungen, Dr. med. Johann Abele, 8e verbeterde oplage, Karl F. Haug Verlag, Heidelberg (Germany) 1991

"Uropathy; A Sure Cure for All Diseases", S.J... Kulkarni, lecture at 20th World Congress of Natural Medicines, 1991 in Madras (India)

"Auto-Urine; The Nectar of Life", B.L. Nalavade, lecture at 20th World Congress of Natural Medicines, 1991 in Madras (India)

All India Directory on Auto Urine Therapy, A.B. Das, Nature Cure and Yoga Research Center, Calcutta (India) 1992

Wonders of Uropathy; Urine Therapy as a Universal Cure , Dr. G. K. Thakkar, Bombay (India) 1992

The Alchemy of Urine; From Witches' Brew to the Golden Elixir; A Diary, Immanu-el Adiv, independent publication, Jerusalem (Israel) 1992

"Urea: Its Possible Role in Auto-Urine Therapy", John Wynhausen, in Shivambu Kalpa Parishad, collected lectures, Goa (India) 1993

Ein ganz besonderer Saft-Urin, Carmen Thomas, vgs verlagsgesellschaft, Köln (Germany) 1993

Die Heilkraft der Eigenharn-Therapie, Ingeborg Allmann, Verlag Dr. Karl Höhn KG, Biberach (Germany) 1993

Index 1. Diseases

Using this index

This index includes most diseases and complaints referred to in the literature on urine therapy studied by the author, and for which, according to this literature, urine therapy has, to a greater or lesser extent, had a beneficial effect. This beneficial effect can range from some relief to total healing, and in general one has to realize that healing is always dependent upon many co-factors.

Under 'General Treatment Suggestions' you will find some guidelines to start treating a certain disease or complaint. In Chapter 4 of this book you will find the precise methods in detail. It is important to realize that there are no strict guidelines for urine therapy. Starting from a general, basic treatment, each individual must find the application of urine therapy which is most appropriate to his needs and, similarly, which other types of treatment should be combined with the urine therapy for the most effective results.

Generally, one can say that in cases of chronic or serious diseases it is useful to fast on urine and water and to have regular massage with, possibly, old urine. This is referred to in this index as 'intensive treatment'. In most cases, even when relatively healthy, this intense form of urine therapy is highly cleansing and health promoting.

Whenever massage is mentioned in these treatment suggestions, it is up to you to choose between massage with old or fresh urine. Here massage generally means just gentle rubbing of urine into the skin or simply applying it to the affected parts.

In the third column, you will find the page(s) where the specific disease or complaint is mentioned in this book.

Where to look in Chapter 4

Application	Page No.
Douching	42
Drinking	38-9
Enemas	41
Eye and eardrops	42
Fasting	39-41
Gargling	42
Homeopathic tincture	43
Urine injections	44
Urine sniffing/Neti	43
Foot and sitbaths	47
Fresh urine rubbings	46
Massage	44,5,46
Scalp and hair massages	47
Urine compresses	46

DISEASES	GENERAL TREATMENT SUGGESTIONS	PAGE(S)
Acne	Washing the face with fresh urine; when possible, cleansing fast.	102
Aging	One glass in the morning as a general tonic, skin massage.	1, 30, 106, 110
AIDS	Intensive treatment including massage and enemas.	ix, 97-102
Allergies	Enemas and injections can be very useful additional treatments; fasting recommended in chronic allergies.	18, 41, 43, 95-7
Amoebas	Drinking, fasting and enemas.	5,91
Amputation	Compresses and drinking.	—
Anemia	Drinking and dietary supplements.	83
Apathy	Drinking.	—
Aphthae	Gargling and dabbing the ulcerous places in the mouth.	—
Appendicitis	Drinking and compresses.	—
Arteriosclerosis	Drinking, massage; sometimes injections are helpful.	66
Arthritis	Drinking, massage and compresses.	97
Asthma	Intensive treatment; injections can be helpful as additional treatment.	21, 65, 80, 81 97
Athlete's foot	Footbath, compress, socks soaked with urine.	47,98
Atrophy	Drinking, massage.	16
Backache	Massage and compresses.	—
Bites	Massage, compress.	83
Bladder problems	Drinking, compresses.	49
Blisters	Compress.	24
Blood pressure (low)	Drinking and dietary adjustments.	—
Blood pressure (high)	Drinking (only small amount) and dietary adjustments.	73,80
Blood vessels (constriction of)	Drinking.	—
Boils	Applying urine on the boils; compresses.	17
Bowel movement	Drinking and enemas.	—
Brain hemorrhage	Drinking, compresses on the head.	16
Bright's disease	Drinking, fasting.	—
Bronchitis	Intensive treatment; injections can be helpful as additional treatment.	83
Bulimia	Drinking.	—
Burns	Massage, compress.	83, 86, 91

DISEASES	GENERAL TREATMENT SUGGESTIONS	PAGE(S)
Energy, low	One glass in the morning as a tonic.	—
Epilepsy	Drinking.	15, 110
Eye problems	Eyebath/drops, putting a few drops in the eyes each time after peeing.	15, 42, 43, 101
– eye infection	Eyebath/drops.	42
– eyesight	Eyebath/drops.	15, 42, 86, 110
Fatigue	Drinking; intensive treatment.	101
Fever	Massage, compresses.	15,86
Flu	Drinking, fasting, massage, gargling, sniffing.	3, 84, 90
Fungus infection	Massage, compress; internal fungus: drinking, enemas.	22, 47, 91
Gall bladder problems	Drinking, fasting and dietary adjustments.	—
Gangrene	Intensive treatment; massage and compresses.	—
Glaucoma	Eyebath/drops.	—
Gonorrhea	Drinking, fasting.	64
Gout	Drinking, compresses; dietary adjustments.	—
Gum disorders	Gargling.	42, 84
Hemorrhoids	Sitbath and compresses; cleansing with fresh urine instead of dry toilet paper.	46, 47
Hair loss	Rubbing the scalp with fresh and old urine.	5, 14, 47, 91
Hay fever	Drinking, eyebaths, sniffing/Neti.	65, 97
Headache	Massage head and neck; compresses.	—
Heart conditions	Drinking, massaging the whole body.	8, 26, 49, 66
Hepatitis	Drinking, fasting, compresses on the liver.	—
Herpes	Drinking, washing the affected spot with urine.	42
HIV	see AIDS.	
Hyperthyroidism	Drinking, compresses on the throat.	—
Hypothyroidism	Drinking, compresses on the throat.	81
Immunity, weakened	One glass in the morning as a tonic; fasting when possible; massage.	92, ff.
Infection	Drinking, compresses.	84, 90

DISEASES	GENERAL TREATMENT SUGGESTIONS	PAGE(S)
Insect bites	Put urine on affected spot; compress.	—
Intestinal problems	Drinking, enemas.	—
Itching	Put urine on affected spots.	15, 97
Jaundice	Drinking, fasting.	15
Joints, pain in the	Massage and compresses.	15
Kaposi Sarcoma	Put urine on affected skin; compresses; intensive treatment; see AIDS.	98
Kidney problems	Drinking, compresses on the kidney areas.	49, 90
Kidney stones	Drinking, compresses on the kidney areas.	89, 91
Leprosy	Intensive treatment; drinking, massage, compresses.	31, 81, 92
Leukemia	Intensive treatment.	—
Leukoderma	Massage, compresses.	—
Limbs, pain in the	Massaging the limbs with (old) urine.	—
Liver infection	Drinking; compresses on the liver.	49
Lung embolism	Drinking.	—
Lymph gland disorders	Drinking, rubbing the affected areas.	89, 101
Malaria	Intensive treatment; drinking, fasting.	32
M.E. (Myalgic Encephalomyelitis)	Intensive treatment; drinking, fasting, enemas, massage.	96
Measles	Drinking; some good results with injections.	18
Meningitis	Intensive treatment; drinking, compresses on the head.	—
Menopause	Drinking.	—
Menstruation problems	Drinking; vaginal douche; compresses on belly.	58
Mental disorder	Drinking.	33, 110
Migraine	Drinking, compresses on the head; enema or injection at the onset of the attack.	15, 97
Mononucleosis	Intensive treatment.	83
Moods	Drinking, massage.	15, 84, 92
Morning sickness	Drinking small amounts of urine, diluted.	18

DISEASES	GENERAL TREATMENT SUGGESTIONS	PAGE(S)
Muscle pain	Massage.	26
Muscular dystrophy	Intensive treatment, massage.	—
Necrosis	Massage, compress.	98
Neurodermitis	Put urine on affected skin areas; compresses; drinking.	—
Nose, blocked	Sniffing/Neti, see also Cold.	43, 89
Obesity	Drinking.	—
Paradontose	Gargling.	42
Paralysis	Drinking, massage.	16
Parasites	Drinking, fasting, enemas.	101
Piles	see Hemorrhoids	15, 47, 81
Pimples	Put urine on the pimples.	88
Plague	Intensive treatment; drinking, fasting.	15
Pneumonia	Intensive treatment; drinking, fasting.	—
Polio	Intensive treatment; drinking, fasting.	—
Possession	Drinking.	—
Prostate disorders	Drinking, compresses on affected area; enemas.	81
Psoriasis	Massage, compresses (with urine mixed with clay); injections can be helpful.	46, 65
Rash	Put urine on affected areas.	45, 46, 86
Rheumatism	Intensive treatment; massage, compresses.	15, 65, 80, 87, 106
Salmonella	Drinking, fasting.	—
Scars	Compresses.	19
Sciatica	Drinking, massage, compresses.	14
Scurvy	Drinking.	15
Sexual potency – decreased	Drinking, massage.	30
Shock	Drinking; when own urine is not available, use urine of someone else.	—

Index 2. General

Other fine products and books for people interested in urine therapy...

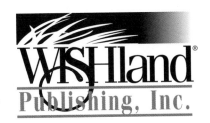

WISHland®
Publishing, Inc.

Name: _____   Phone: _____

Address: _____

City: _____ State: _____ Zip: _____

P.O. Box 41504
Mesa, Arizona 85274
(480) 922-8511
Fax: (480) 443-3386

Item #	Description	Cost	Total
W1516	**The Golden Fountain** *by Coen Van Der Kroon*	$14.95	
W1500	**Your Own Perfect Medicine** *by Martha Christy* *(Complete book on the medical and clinical research on urine therapy - our best seller!)*	$19.95	
W1501	**The Water of Life** *by John Armstrong* *(Great testimonial reading!)*	$11.95	
W1900	**Simple Diagnostic Tests You Can Do At Home** *(Provides the information to interpret the chemstrips and pH paper readings)*	$9.95	
W1907	**pH Papers** *(test the acidity or alkalinity of your urine)*	$15.95	
W1902	**Chemstrips** for urine testing	$15.99	
W1502	**Scientific Validation of Urine Therapy** *by Martha Christy* (Audio Tape)	$11.00	
W1513	**101 Ways to Use Your Own Perfect Medicine** (Audio Tape)	$11.00	
W1512	**How to Fast on Your Own Perfect Medicine** (Audio Tape)	$15.00	
W1504	**Introduction to Urine Therapy** *an interview with Martha Christy* (Audio Tape)	$11.00	
W1503	**You're in Good Health** (Testimonial Tape)	$11.00	
	Shipping & Handling: All orders over $35.00 are shipped free of charge. Orders under $35.00 please add $5.00		
	Foreign Orders add $35.00 to charges, orders to Canada add $25.00		
	Arizona Residents only - Add 7.5% Sales Tax		
	TOTAL AMOUNT ENCLOSED:		

To order by phone, call 480-922-8511, or mail to Wishland Publishing, P.O. Box 41504, Mesa, AZ 85274

Please Charge my Credit Card # _____ *Exp. Date:* _____

Signature: _____

Other fine products and books for people interested in urine therapy...

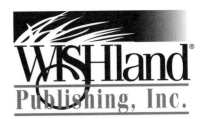

WISHland Publishing, Inc.

Name: _____ Phone: _____

Address: _____

City: _____ State: _____ Zip: _____

P.O. Box 41504
Mesa, Arizona 85274
(480) 922-8511
Fax: (480) 443-3386

Item #	Description	Cost	Total
W1516	**The Golden Fountain** *by Coen Van Der Kroon*	$14.95	
W1500	**Your Own Perfect Medicine** *by Martha Christy*	$19.95	
	(Complete book on the medical and clinical research on urine therapy - our best seller!)		
W1501	**The Water of Life** *by John Armstrong*	$11.95	
	(Great testimonial reading!)		
W1900	**Simple Diagnostic Tests You Can Do At Home**	$9.95	
	(Provides the information to interpret the chemstrips and pH paper readings)		
W1907	**pH Papers** *(test the acidity or alkalinity of your urine)*	$15.95	
W1902	**Chemstrips** for urine testing	$15.99	
W1502	**Scientific Validation of Urine Therapy** *by Martha Christy* (Audio Tape)	$11.00	
W1513	**101 Ways to Use Your Own Perfect Medicine** (Audio Tape)	$11.00	
W1512	**How to Fast on Your Own Perfect Medicine** (Audio Tape)	$15.00	
W1504	**Introduction to Urine Therapy** *an interview with Martha Christy* (Audio Tape)	$11.00	
W1503	**You're in Good Health** (Testimonial Tape)	$11.00	
	Shipping & Handling:		
	All orders over $35.00 are shipped free of charge. Orders under $35.00 please add $5.00		
	Foreign Orders add $35.00 to charges, orders to Canada add $25.00		
	Arizona Residents only - Add 7.5% Sales Tax		
	TOTAL AMOUNT ENCLOSED:		

To order by phone, call 480-922-8511, or mail to Wishland Publishing, P.O. Box 41504, Mesa, AZ 85274

Please Charge my Credit Card # _____ *Exp. Date:* _____

Signature: _____